OUT OF TH
HOW

Naming your baby is a decision that will last a life-time. You need a reliable reference that will give you a selection of boys' and girls' names to fit your taste, lifestyle, and family traditions. *10,000 Names for Your Baby*—now updated with thousands of *new* choices—makes finding the perfect name easier than ever. Don't miss:

- Place names for boys and girls—TARA, JAMAICA, DAKOTA, DENVER
- Surnames for first names—MADISON, PALMER, HARPER, TAYLOR
- Names from nature—LARK, PEARL, JAY, SAGE
- Biblical names—TAMAR, HANNAH, GABRIEL, ISAIAH
- Virtue or value names—HONOR, MERCY, FORTUNE, BLISS
- Names from mythology—DAPHNE, THEA, GARETH, THOR
  . . . and so much more!

GREAT BABY NAME IDEAS
ADVICE YOU CAN TRUST
10,000 NAMES FOR YOUR BABY

10,000 NAMES
FOR YOUR BABY

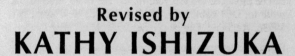

Revised by
KATHY ISHIZUKA

A Dell Book

Published by
Dell Publishing
a division of
Random House, Inc.
1540 Broadway
New York, New York 10036

ISBN: 0-440-22336-9

Printed in the United States of America

Published simultaneously in Canada

May 1997

OPM 21 20 19 18 17 16 15 14 13

Infant Joy

'I have no name—
I am but two days old.'
What shall I call thee?
'I happy am,
Joy is my name.'
Sweet joy befall thee!

Pretty joy!
Sweet joy but two days old—
Sweet joy I call thee,
Thou dost smile,
I sing the while—
Sweet joy befall thee!

William Blake

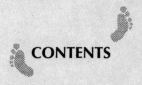

CONTENTS

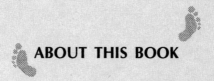

ABOUT THIS BOOK

This fully updated edition contains more than 11,400 names, double the entries of the previous volume. You will find complete descriptions of all the traditional European names, as well as African, Asian, Arabic, Latino, and American Indian, among others. Here too are all the hottest contemporary names, including place names, surnames, and invented names.

The expanded entries contain the word's origin, definition, and, wherever necessary, a pronunciation guide. Also listed are notable namesakes, among them: scientists, writers, entertainment figures, biblical characters and saints, political and business leaders, and athletes. In addition many entries feature anecdotal information on mythological, biblical, historical, or literary associations related to that name.

You will also find a horoscope section, completely revised to enlighten your search for the perfect name for your baby. Enjoy!

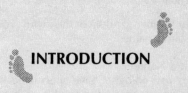

INTRODUCTION

How We Choose Names

Parents-to-be may be overwhelmed by the responsibility of naming their baby. It is, after all, their first formal act as parents, and subject to the scrutiny of family, friends, and community. A name can proclaim parents' hopes for their child and how they define themselves as a family. Your personal, religious, and cultural identity can be measured, in part, by the name you give your child. Understanding the importance of the task before them, many parents feel overwhelmed because in our culture there are no guidelines and few traditions concerning the naming of babies. What has been described as your first gift to your child is a personal choice, and is often decided in what may seem to be an arbitrary manner.

Despite the private nature of your decision, you will undoubtedly be subjected to many opinions along the way. Even before Aunt Edna (or another relative) puts in her two cents, you will probably encounter some material on the subject. Popular baby-name books abound. Most are references of a general sort; however, there are also books that recommend celebrity names, names of soap opera characters, and names scientifically measured for professional and personal success. One best-selling book defines every possible subgroup of names, which are cleverly headed and classified according to style. Parents can choose, in menu fashion, which style they aspire to. Most recent on the market is a board game devised for selecting a name, step-by-step.

While a good baby-name reference (like the one you have in your hands) can help guide you in your quest, your final choice remains a personal one. Does the name sound pleasing? Is it meaningful? Does it honor your family? Only you can make these decisions for yourself and your child. So relax, trust your instincts, and savor the joyful process of discovering your child's name.

What's in a Name?

For years psychologists have speculated that a person's first name can somehow influence his or her life. Here are some recent findings on the significance of names.

Feminine Names: A widely published British study seemed to confirm that girls with feminine names like Lucy and Rose did indeed have more girlish personalities. However, this result may have had more to do with the traditional parents who named them. Another study on women with masculine names (Dean, Randy, etc.) revealed that they were no more likely to be unfeminine than women named Deborah or Elizabeth. Yet another study compares the relationship between women's names and corporate hiring. It contends that, at least in white-collar circles, there is prejudice against sexy names—in other words, a Crystal may be passed over for promotion in favor of an Amanda.

Children and Their Names: New research in this area has debunked a widely accepted theory that academic achievement and "social competence" are linked to the popularity of a child's name—in other words, that Ashley and Michael would have more friends and be more favorably graded by teachers than their less popularly named peers, such as Agnes and Myron. The researchers concluded that names were "not at all related" to success in these areas. They also found that, in relationships, a person's name is not an important issue once you get to know him or her well, at which point other characteristics become more influential.

Unusual Names: Several older studies have led us to believe that people with unusual names are more likely to be unpopular or to even show signs of psychosis. More recent research, however, seems to indicate that on written personality tests, unusually named people have the same kinds of personalities as more conventionally named ones. The psychologists who conducted the study stated, "Neither men nor women appear to be at a psychological disadvantage as a result of having an unusual or sexually ambiguous name." Clearly, more research is indicated in this area—particularly the examination of parents who give their children unusual names.

Some Popular Categories of Names

While this book does not promote baby-naming trends, there are specific name types that might be of interest to list here. At any rate, it might aid your decision-making process by helping you to think in terms of categories of names.

Ethnic Names: Perhaps the most striking aspect of baby naming today is the growing popularity of ethnic names. Many of these names, once considered rare or very unusual, are commonly heard in playgrounds across the country and regularly appear in popular baby-name books.

In an atmosphere of increased ethnic awareness, many families are making their own very strong, personal statement by giving their children names that proclaim their ethnic and cultural identity. Multiculturalism is not just a passing issue, but an indicator of the changing face of America; recent demographics estimate that minorities will constitute half of the total U.S. population by the year 2050.

A related phenomenon is the rise in interracial families, which has also impacted baby naming. The dual ethnicity of this generation is expressed in their colorful names: Tamika O'Shawnessy (African-American/Irish); Keiji Drysdale (Scottish/Japanese American); Pontius Sun Jung (Korean/Mexican/Irish/Chinese). Many baby-name books, including the previous edition of this one, actually warn against combining names of different ethnic groups or cultures. However, contemporary families are defying this outdated notion in increasing numbers.

Foreign-language names are not solely reserved for children of those ethnic groups. Many of these beautiful names are adopted cross-culturally, particularly Hawaiian names, some of which are used so often that they are approaching classic status.

You will find ethnic names scattered throughout this updated edition—there are far too many to list all of them here. If you would like to further your research, there are now available several references devoted to personal names of specific ethnic groups and cultures. Check your local library or bookseller.

Place Names: This is a rich group of names, including both proper names (Boston, India) and descriptive terms (Clifford, Dale). The following list is only a small sampling of possibilities. You can choose the name of a place significant to you, a hometown or state, a foreign place name or term reflecting your ancestral roots, the baby's birthplace, or even the place where she or he was conceived. Of course, you may also choose a place name simply because it sounds pleasant to you and has a nice meaning. We know of a couple who did just that, plucking a faraway place name from an atlas and bestowing it on their daughter, who, as far as we know, is still pleased with her unique, melodic name.

Girls

Arcadia	Iona	Nila
Asia	Jamaica	Oceania
Boston	Jordan	Paris
Caledonia	Juniata	Savannah
Catalina	Kenya	Sevilla
China	Kiona	Shannon
Dakota	Kyle	Sienna
Elysia	Lourdes	Tara
Florida	Montana	Tiberia
Glenna	Nara	Tosca
Hadley	Nevada	Whitney
India		

Boys

Brendan	Haden	Morgan
Brett	Holland	Nash
Cashel	Hudson	Nazareth
Clifford	Jordan	Ogden
Clyde	Keith	Ralston
Dakota	Kent	Ramsey
Dale	Kyle	Roman
Dallas	Lane	Shannon
Dean	Lincoln	Stanford
Denholm	Marsden	Tyrone
Denver	Mead	Wesley
Granville	Montana	

Surnames: Surnames or family names were traditionally used for boys' first names, but today they are popular choices for both sexes. Parents may choose to honor the mother's family by selecting her family name as a first or middle name.

Below is a brief listing of the more popular surnames that can serve as first names for either sex. Family sources can help you in researching your own name, or you can check the reference section of the library, where you should find several volumes on surnames, their origin and meaning.

Blake	Harper	Potter
Campbell	Kelly	Quinn
Carson	MacKenzie	Reed
Carter	Madison	Riley
Cassidy	Miller	Sawyer
Chaney	Palmer	Shelby
Chapin	Parker	Sheridan
Grayson	Payton/Peyton	Taylor

Names from Nature: At first glance, these names may have a "back-to-nature," retro-seventies connotation for you. But examine the list and you will find many beautiful, melodic names, as well as many classics, such as Todd and Susan (meaning fox and lily, respectively), which you might not have thought of as nature names.

Girls

Acacia	Ivie/Ivy	Morela
Alyssa	Jade	Olivia
Amber	Kai	Oprah
Ayla	Kleantha	Pala
Beryl	Lani	Paloma
Blossom	Lark	Pearl
Brooke	Laurel	Rosalind
Calandra	Leona	Ruby
Calla	Leotie	Rue
Columbia	Lian	Susan
Concha	Linnea	Tabitha
Coral	Luna	Ulma
Doe	Mahina	Violet
Ebony	Margaret	Willow
Eirlys	Maris	Wren
Gemma	Marjani	Yuki
Hamelia	Mavis	Zipporah
Hana		

Boys

Alder	Frazier	Nevada
Barend/Berend	Hart	Oren
Bertram	Hawthorne	Orson
Beryl	Herschel	Peregrine
Birch	Hickory	Raven
Brooks	Jaafar	Ravi
Buck	Jasper	Robin
Callum/Colm	Jay	Sage
Cedar	Kai	Sierra
Chayton	Lark	Silas/Silvano
Colt	Leonard	Sky
Corbin	Marsh	Storm
Eben	Merle	Todd
Ferris	Merlin	Verne/Vernon
Forrest	Mesa	

Biblical Names: The tradition of biblical names has endured through the years, with the less-common names—such as Ketura and Isaiah—growing in popularity.

Girls

Abigail	Eve	Mary (Mari,
Bethany	Hannah	Maria, etc.)
Carmel	Jordan	Moriah
Deborah	Judith	Naomi
Delilah	Keshia	Rachel
Dinah	Ketura	Rebecca
Eden	Leah	Ruth
Elizabeth	Martha	Tamar
Esther		

Boys

Aaron	Benjamin	Gabriel
Abner	Daniel	Isaac
Abraham	Darius	Isaiah
Adam	Demetrius	Jacob
Andrew	Elijah	James
Bartholomew	Ephraim	Jeremiah

Joel	Matthew	Philip
John	Micah	Seth
Jonah	Noah	Thaddeus
Josiah	Paul	Thomas
Luke	Peter	Zachariah
Mark		

Virtue or Value Names: This interesting group is based on the virtue names favored by the Puritans in the 1600s. We have expanded the category to include value words that are used to name modern-day children.

Both sexes

Blessing	Honor	Peace
Bliss	Hope	Prosper
Charity	Justice	Prudence
Comfort	Love	Purity
Constant	Loyal	Strong
Courage	Mercy	Temperance
Devotion	Mirth	True, Truly
Fortune	Modesto, Modesty	Virtue
Harmony	Patience, Patient	Welcome

Names from Mythology: On the following list you'll find names from world mythology in addition to the classical characters.

Girls

Artemisia	Dione	Olympia
Astraea	Evadne	Pandora
Aurora	Gaea	Penelope
Basilia	Helen	Phoebe
Camilla	Hina	Raven
Cassandra	Indra	Rhea
Chandra	Iris	Rhiannon
Clementine	Kali	Selena
Clio	Latonia	Thalia
Danae	Maeve	Thea
Daphne	Maia	Venus
Demetria	Minerva	

Boys

Adonis	Griffin	Nestor
Alvis	Hermes	Orion
Andros	Indra	Ossian
Apollo	Janus	Sol
Arthur	Jason	Thor
Gareth	Lancelot	Zeus

Classic Names: Many parents remain conservative when choosing a name for their children. One geographer's research found that the three most popular boys' names in New England today—John, William, and James—were the same top three in 1790.

There are far too many classic names to list here; most are described in detail in the A-to-Z section. For select common names—including Michael, John, and Mary—there are reference books devoted to that name, including its history and exhaustive lists of famous namesakes. Check your local library or bookseller.

Customized Names: Perhaps you've already chosen a name, but want to change it in some way to make it uniquely yours. You can achieve this with an alternate spelling or variant of the name—numerous possibilities follow main entries in this book, or you can create your own. Keep in mind, however, that your child will have to monitor its correct spelling.

Invented Names: With a bit of thought and imagination you can create a truly unique name for your child. You can combine syllables or names, for example: Albert and Victoria = Altoria. The first name of Irita van Doren, literary editor, was coined by her mother from Ida and Marguerite. Acronyms have also been used to create names, as have anagrams, in which letters of a significant word are scrambled.

Naming No-Nos
—Humorous names. Robin Banks, Lily White, Rusty Hammer, Rose Bush, and the like.
—"Junior." Some believe it connotes sissiness or youthfulness. One recent study proves that the diminutive moniker is indeed a psychological disadvantage.

—Alliteration. For example: Bethany Brooke Boorstin.
—Rhyming first and last names.
—Embarrassing initials. Do they spell a word?

Ten Considerations When Choosing a Name

1) Start early. Broach the issue with your partner soon; remember, this is a joint decision that will naturally take some time to negotiate. Some parents may feel uncomfortable with deciding on a name very early, but at least you can get an idea of your partner's feelings on the subject, and you can make clear your own criteria for choosing a name. Are you looking for a name of a certain meaning; do you want it to reflect your ethnic heritage; are trendy names completely out of the question?

If you are a "list" sort of person, start making one now.

2) Cultural, ethnic, or religious considerations. Various cultures have specific naming traditions you may wish to follow. For example, in Jewish culture it is unlucky to name a baby after a living relative, and Catholics traditionally name children after saints. In certain African cultures, names pay homage to ancestors or indicate the time of the child's birth, the day, or the season. If you would like to learn more about your own traditions, begin by consulting your family.

3) Would you like to honor a family member? You can accomplish this with either a first or middle name. Make this decision before you actually begin looking for a name.

4) Sound and rhythm. Once you've made some selections, repeat the name out loud and see how it sounds to you.

5) The baby's last name. Will it automatically be the father's family name? Today this may be an issue for some parents, who might choose a hyphenated last name (mother's-father's last name), incorporate the mother's family name as a middle name, or choose to use the mother's last name alone. Your child's first name should combine harmoniously with his last. Again, this is a matter of personal taste. Write down the full name to see how it looks and sound it out.

6) Meaning. Use this book to research the meaning of the name, as well as any associations with famous namesakes.

7) Imagine the name being used in a variety of circumstances. Cute or very stylish names may be considered less appropriate later in your child's life.

8) Nicknames. Imagine all the possible nicknames that can be derived from your choice and decide whether you and your child could live with them.

9) Spelling. An unusual name or spelling stands out as unique; however, you should also consider the fact that your child will have to monitor its correct spelling and pronunciation throughout his or her life.

10) Don't make a final decision until you actually see your baby. Take a short list to the hospital. And remember that doctors can make mistakes in predicting the sex of the child, so have two sets of names, just in case.

NAMES FOR BOYS

NAMES FOR BOYS

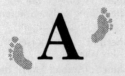

Aaron: (Hebrew) "light; high mountain." Biblical: the brother of Moses, considered to be the founder of the Jewish priesthood. Aaron Copland, American composer.
Also: **Aeron, Aren, Aron.**

Abbot: (Hebrew) "father."
Also: **Abbott.**

Abdul, Abdullah: (Arabic) "Servant of the Lord."
Also: **Abdiel, Abdulla.**

Abe, Abie: see Abraham.

Abel: (Hebrew) "breath." Biblical: the second son of Adam and Eve, slain by his brother Cain. Abel Gance, film director (1889–1981).

Abelard: (Teutonic) "resolute; ambitious."

Abner: (Hebrew) "of light; bright." Biblical: cousin of Saul.
Also: **Ab, Abbie, Avner.**

Abraham: (Hebrew) "father of many; exalted father." Biblical: founder figure in both Jewish and Christian tradition. Abraham Lincoln, 16th U. S. President.
Also: **Abe, Abie, Abram, Avram, Bram, Ibrahim.**

Abram: see Abraham.

Absalom: (Hebrew) "father of peace." Biblical: son of King David.

Ace: (Latin) "unity."

Ackerly: (Old English) "dweller at the acre meadow."

Ackley: (Old English) "dweller at the oak-tree meadow."

Adair: (Celtic) "from the oak-tree ford."

Adal: (Teutonic) "noble."
Also: **Adel.**

Adalard: see Adelard.

Adalbert: see Albert.

Adam: (Hebrew) "red earth; man of earth." The biblical "first man."
Also: **Adamah, Adami, Adams, Adamson, Addam.** See also Adin.

Adar: (Hebrew) "noble." In the Jewish calendar, one of the spring months.

Addis: (Anglo-Saxon) "axe wielder."

Addison: (Anglo-Saxon) "Adam's descendant."

Adelard: (Teutonic) "resolute; noble."
Also: **Adalard.**

Aden: *see* Aidan.

Adil: (Swahili) "just."

Adin: (Hebrew) "voluptuous; sensual."

Adir: (Hebrew) "mighty; glorious."

Adlai: (Hebrew) "my ornament." Adlai Stevenson, American politician.
Also: **Adley.**

Adler: (Old German) "eagle."
Also: **Adlar.**

Adnan: (Arabic) "heaven."

Adney: (Old English) "dweller on the noble one's island."

Adolfo: (Teutonic) "noble wolf."
Also: **Adolph, Adolphe, Adolphus, Dolph.**

Adon: (Phoenician) "lord." Adonal Foyle, basketball player.

Adonis: (Greek) "handsome." Mythology: in Greek myth, the handsome shepherd loved by both Aphrodite and Persephone.

Adrian: (Latin) "dark; from Adria." Name of a Roman emperor and several popes. Adrian Lyne, film director.
Also: **Adriano, Adrien (Fr), Hadrian.**

Adriel: (Hebrew) "from God's congregation."

Aelwyn: *see* Alvin.

Aeneas: (Greek) "the praised one." In the *Aeneid* Aeneas was the Trojan hero whose descendants founded Rome.

Aeron: (Welsh) "fruit; berry."

Africa: (Gaelic) "pleasant." The origin of the name of the continent is unclear.

Agur: (Hebrew) "gatherer."

Ahab: (Hebrew) "uncle." Biblical: king of Israel, enemy of the prophet Elijah.

Ahern: (Celtic) "horse lord."
Also: **Ahearn.**

Ahmed: (Arabic) "most highly praised." Ahmed III, sultan of the Ottoman Empire; Ahmad Rashad, sportscaster.
Also: **Ahmad, Amad.**

Ahmik: (American Indian) "the beaver, symbol of skill."

Ahsan: (Arabic) "charity."

Aidan: (Irish/Gaelic) "little fire." Aidan Quinn, actor.
Also: **Aden, Aiden.**

Aiken: (Anglo-Saxon) "oaken."

Ainsley: (Old English) "of a nearby meadow."
Also: **Ainslie.**

Akbar: (Arabic) "great." Akbar, emperor of India.

Aki: (ah-KEE) (Japanese) "autumn; bright." Akira Kurosawa, film director; Akio Morita, founder, Sony Corporation.

Al: short form of names beginning Al-.

Alan: (Celtic) "handsome; harmony."
Also: **Alain, Aland, Allain,**

Allan, Allayne, Allen, Alleyn, Allyn.

Aland: *see* Alan.

Alaric: (Teutonic) "ruler of all." Alaric I, king of the Visigoths.
Also: **Alarick, Rich, Richie, Rick, Ulric, Ulrich, Ulrick.**

Alastair: a form of Alexander.
Also: **Alistair, Allister.**

Alban: (Latin) "white." St. Alban was the first British martyr, killed in AD 209 for sheltering persecuted Christians.
Also: **Alben, Albin, Alva.**

Albern: (Old English) "noble warrior."

Albert: (Teutonic) "noble and bright." Prince Albert, husband of Queen Victoria.
Also: **Adalard, Adalbert, Adelard, Al, Alberto, Albrecht, Bert, Bertie, Elbert, Ethelbert.**

Albion: *see* Aubin.

Alcott: (Celtic) "from the stone cottage."
Also: **Alcot.**

Alden: (Anglo-Saxon) "old friend." Neil Alden Armstrong, first astronaut to walk on the moon.
Also: **Al, Aldin, Aldwin, Alwin.**

Alder: (Teutonic) "the alder tree."

Aldo: (Teutonic) "rich."

Aldous: (Teutonic) "old; wise." Aldous Huxley, novelist (1894–1964).
Also: **Aldis, Aldus.**

Aldrich: (Teutonic) "king."
Also: **Alderic, Aldric.**

Aldridge: *see* Aldrich.

Alec, Alex: *see* Alexander.

Aled: (Welsh) a Welsh place name used as a first name.

Aleron: (Middle Latin) "eagle."

Alexander: (Greek) "protector of men." Alexander the Great.
Also: **Al, Alastair, Alec, Aleck, Alejandro (Sp), Aleksandr (Russ), Aleksy, Alessandro (It), Alex, Alexandre (Fr), Alexis, Alick, Alistair, Allister, Ally, Lex, Sander, Sandor (Hung), Sandy, Saunders, Zander.**

Alfonso: *see* Alphonse.

Alford: (Old English) "the old ford or river crossing."

Alfred: (Anglo-Saxon) "wise as an elf." Alfred, king of England. Alfred Nobel, inventor of dynamite.
Also: **Al, Alf, Alfeo, Alfie, Alfredo, Alfy.**

Alger: (Anglo-Saxon) "spearman."
Also: **Algar.**

Algernon: (French) "bearded." Algernon Blackwood, author.
Also: **Al, Algie, Algy.**

Ali: (Arabic) "noble; great."

Alistair: *see* Alexander.

Allan: *see* Alan.

Allard: (Old English) "sacred and brave."
Also: **Alard.**

Allison: (English) "Alice's son." Allison Danzig, sportswriter.

Almeric: (Teutonic) "work; rule."
Also: **Almery, Awly.**

Alon: (Hebrew) "oak tree."
Also: **Allon.**

Alonzo: Spanish form of Alphonse.

Aloysius: *see* Lewis.

Alphonse: (Teutonic) "prepared for battle."
Also: **Alfonso, Alonzo, Alphonso.**

Alpin: (Pictish-Scottish) "blond one."

Alroy: (Irish Gaelic) "red-haired youth."

Altman: (Old German) "old, wise man."

Alton: (Anglo-Saxon) "dweller at the old town or estate." Alton Ellis, singer.
Also: **Alston, Elton.**

Alva: (Latin) "white." Thomas Alva Edison, inventor.
Also: **Alvah.**

Alvah: (Hebrew) "exalted one."

Alvern: (Latin) "of the springtime."

Alvin: (Teutonic) "friend of all." Alvin Ailey, choreographer. Elvin Bishop, musician.
Also: **Aelwyn, Alvan, Alvino (Sp), Alwin, Alwyn.**

Alvis: (Old Norse) "all-wise." In Norse mythology, the suitor of Thor's daughter.
Also: **Elvis.**

Alworth: (Teutonic) "esteemed by all."

Amadeo: (Latin/Spanish) "He who loves God." Amadeo

P. Gianini, founder, Bank of America.
Also: **Amadeus.**

Amal: (Arabic) "hope." (Hebrew) "work."

Amand: (French) "worthy of love."

Amani: (Swahili) "peace."

Amara: (Sanskrit) "immortal."

Amasa: (Hebrew) "burden bearer." Amasa Stone, financier.

Ambert: (Teutonic) "shining light; bright."

Ambler: (English) "stable keeper."

Ambrose: (Greek) "belonging to the immortals." Ambrose Bierce, American writer.

Amery: *see* Amory.

Amiel: (Hebrew) "my nation belongs to God."

Amis: (Latin) origin obscure.
Also: **Ames.**

Ammon: (Egyptian) the ancient Egyptian sun god.

Amon: (Hebrew) "educator, architect."

Amory: (English) "brave; powerful." (Latin) "affectionate."
Also: **Amary, Amery.**

Amos: (Hebrew) "bearer of a burden." Biblical: the Book of Amos.

Amund: (Scandinavian) "divine protector."

An: (Chinese/Vietnamese) "peace; peaceful." An Wang, founder, Wang Laboratories.

Anastatius: (Greek) "one who is reborn."
Also: **Anastas, Anastasius.**

Anatole: (Greek) "of the east."
Also: **Anatol.**

Anders: Scandinavian form of Andrew.
Also: **Anderson.**

Andrei: *see* Andrew. Andrei Sakharov, Nobel physicist.

Andrew: (Greek) "manly." Biblical: one of the twelve apostles, brother of Simon Peter. St. Andrew, patron saint of Scotland and Russia.
Also: **Anders (Scan), Andre (Fr), Andreas, Andrei (Slavic), Andreo, Andres (Sp), Andrien, Andros, Andy, Drew.**

Andy: *see* Andrew.

Aneurin, Aneirin: (Welsh) "little one of pure gold." Aneurin Bevan, founder of Britain's National Health Service.
Also: **Neirin, Nye.**

Ang: (Chinese) "spirited." Traditionally combined with a second name. Ang Lee, film-maker.

Angel, Angelo: (Greek) "saintly." Angel Cordero, jockey.
Also: **Angelo.**

Angus: (Celtic) "exceptional; outstanding." The name of a Scottish county.
Also: **Gus.**

Angwyn: (Welsh) "handsome."
Also: **Angwen.**

Annan: (Celtic) "from the stream."

Anoki: (American Indian) "actor."

Anscom: (Old English) "dweller in the valley of the awe-inspiring one."

Ansel: (Old French) "adherent of a nobleman." Ansel Adams, photographer. *See also* Anselm.

Anselm: (Teutonic) "divine helmet of God." Saint Anselm of Canterbury.
Also: **Ansel, Anzelm.**

Ansley: (Old English) "from the awe-inspiring one's pasture meadow."

Anson: (Anglo-Saxon) "the son of Ann."

Anstice: (Greek) "resurrected one."

Anthony: (Latin) "of inestimable worth." Saint Anthony, father of Christian monasticism.
Also: **Antoine (Fr), Anton (Slavic), Antoni, Antonio (It), Antony, Tony.**

Anton, Antonio: *see* Anthony. Anton Chekhov, dramatist.

Anwar: (Arabic) "luminous." Anwar Sadat, Egyptian president, winner of the Nobel Peace Prize.

Anwell: (Welsh-Celtic) "beloved or dear one."
Also: **Anwyl.**

Anyon: (Welsh-Celtic) "anvil."

Apollo: (Greek) the Greek and

Roman god of light, music, and poetry.
Also: **Apolinar.**

Aquilino: (Latin) "eagle."

Archard: (Anglo-French-German) "sacred, powerful."

Archer: (Old English) "bowman." *See also* Archibald.

Archibald: (Teutonic) "truly bold; bold archer." Archibald MacLeish, writer.
Also: **Archer, Archie, Archy.**

Archie, Archy: *see* Archibald.

Arden: (Latin) "fervent; eager and sincere."
Also: **Ardon.**

Ardley: (Old English) "from the home-lover's meadow."

Aren: a form of Aaron.

Arfon: a Welsh place name.

Argentino: (Latin) "silvery."

Argus: (Greek) "watchful; vigilant."
Also: **Gus.**

Argyle: (Scotch Gaelic) "from the land of the Gaels; an Irishman."

Ari: (Hebrew) "lion." (Norse) "eagle."

Aric: (Old English) "sacred ruler."
Also: **Arik.**

Ariel: (Hebrew) "lion of God." Ariel Sharon, Israeli statesman.
Also: **Arel, Arie.**

Aries: (Latin) "a ram."

Arion: (Greek) "esteemed." Mythology: Arion was a Greek poet and musician.

Arledge: (Old English) "dweller at rabbit lake."

Arlen: (Irish Gaelic) "pledge."
Also: **Arlan.**

Arlie: *see* Harley.

Arlo: (Latin) "the barberry bush." Arlo Guthrie, singer.

Armand, Armin, Armond: *see* Herman. Armand Hammer, businessman, philanthropist.

Armistead: (Teutonic) "a place of arms." Armistead Maupin, writer.

Armstrong: (Old English) "with a strong arm."

Arnall: (Old German) "eagle; gracious."

Arnaud: variant of Arnold.

Arnett: (Old Franco-English) "little eagle."

Arney: (Old German) "eagle."

Arnold: (Teutonic) "strong as an eagle."
Also: **Arnaldo, Arnaud, Arne, Arnie, Arno.**

Arnot: (Old Franco-German) "little eagle."

Arsenio: (Greek) "virile, masculine." Arsenio Hall, television personality.
Also: **Arsen, Arsene (Fr), Arsenius.**

Artemas: (Greek) "gift of Artemis." Artemas Ward, Revolutionary War general.
Also: **Artemio, Artemus.**

Arthur: (Celtic) "strong as a rock." King Arthur, legendary British monarch of the 6th century.
Also: **Art, Arte, Artie, Artur (Pol), Arturo (Sp).**

Arturo: *see* Arthur.

Arundel: (Old English) "dweller at the eagle dell."

Arval: (Latin) "wept over." Also: **Arvel.**

Arvin: (Teutonic) "a friend of the people." Also: **Arv, Arvie, Arvy.**

Arwel: (Welsh) "prominent."

Asa: (Hebrew) "healer." Biblical: the king of Judah.

Asad: (Islamic) "lion."

Ascot: (Old English) "dweller at the east cottage."

Ash: (Old English) "ash tree." Also: a short form of names beginning Ash-.

Ashburn: (Old English) "dweller at the ash-tree stream."

Ashby: (Old English) "ash-tree farm."

Asher: (Hebrew) "fortunate." Biblical: the son of Jacob. Asher Durand, painter.

Ashford: (Old English) "dweller at the ash-tree ford."

Ashley: (Old English) "dweller in the ash-tree meadow." Also: **Lee.**

Ashlin: (Old English) "dweller at the ash-tree pool."

Ashton: (Old English) "dweller at the ash-tree farm."

Athan: (Greek) "immortal."

Athelstan: (Old English) "noble stone." Athelstan, king of Wessex.

Athens: (Greek) the Greek goddess of wisdom.

Atherton: (Old English) "dweller at the spring farm."

Athol: a Scottish place name of unknown meaning. Athol Fugard, South African playwright.

Atley: (Old English) "dweller at the meadow."

Atticus: Atticus Finch, Southern lawyer of *To Kill a Mockingbird* (1960), by Harper Lee.

Atwater: (Old English) "dweller at the water."

Atwell: (Old English) "dweller at the spring."

Atwood: (Old English) "dweller at the forest."

Atworth: (Old English) "dweller at the farmstead."

Auberon: *see* Aubrey.

Aubin: (Latin) "fair, white." Also: **Albion, Aubyn.**

Aubrey: (Teutonic) "elf-ruler." Aubrey Beardsley, English illustrator. Also: **Auberon, Aubry.**

Auden: (English) "old friend." Audie Murphy, war hero, actor.

August: (Latin) "exalted." St. Augustine; August Wilson, dramatist. Also: **Augie, Augustin, Augustine, Augusto, Augustus, Austen, Austin, Gus, Gustane, Gustin.**

Augustine: *see* August.

Aurelio: (Spanish) "golden." Also: **Aurelius, Auren, Oriel, Oriole.**

Aurick: *see* Warrick.

Austin: *see* August.

Avalon: (Celtic) In legend, the Isle of Souls, an earthly paradise somewhere in the Western seas.

Avenall: (Old French) "dweller at the oat field."

Averill: (Anglo-Saxon) "boar-like; of April." Averell Harriman, statesman.
Also: **Averil.**

Avery: (Anglo-Saxon) "ruler of the elves." Avery Brundage, Olympic sports figure.

Avner: variant of Abner.

Avram: *see* Abraham.

Axel: Scandinavian form of Absalom.

Axton: (Old English) "sword wielder's stone."

Aylmer: *see* Elmer.

Aylward: (Old English) "awe-inspiring guardian."

Aylworth: (Old English) "awe-inspiring one's farmstead."

Aymon: French variant of Raymond.

Aziel: (Hebrew) "whom God strengthens."
Also: **Azriel.**

B

Bai: (Chinese) "cypress." Traditionally combined with a second name.

Bailey: (Teutonic) "bailiff."
Also: **Bayley.**

Bainbridge: (Old English) "bridge over white water."

Baird: (Celtic) "the minstrel."
Also: **Bard.**

Balder: (Old English) "bold army."

Baldric: (Teutonic) "bold or princely ruler."

Baldwin: (Teutonic) "bold, noble friend."

Balfour: (Pictish-Gaelic) "from the pasture place."

Ballard: (Old German) "bold, strong."

Balor: (Old French) "bale maker."

Balthasar: (Greek) "may the Lord protect the king."
Also: **Baltasar.**

Bancroft: (Anglo-Saxon) "from the bean field." Ban (Byron Bancroft) Johnson, president of baseball's American League.

Banning: (Irish Gaelic) "little blond one."
Also: **Bannon.**

Bannister: (English) "basketmaker."

Barbour: (Old English) "a barber."
Also: **Barber.**

Barclay: *see* Berkeley.

Bard: *see* Baird.

Bardrick: (Old English) "axe ruler."

Barend: (Dutch) "bear."
Also: **Berend.**

Barker: (Scandinavian) "a bark stripper."

Barlow: (Old English) "dweller at the bare hill."

Barnaby: (Hebrew) "son of prophecy or consolation." Also: **Barnabas, Barnett, Barney.**

Barnard: *see* Bernard.

Barnett: (Old English) "nobleman; leader." Barnett Newman, artist.

Barney: *see* Barnaby, Baruch, Bernard.

Barnum: (Old English) "nobleman's home." Barnum Brown, 19th-century dinosaur hunter.

Baron: (Teutonic) "of noble blood." Barron G. Collier, advertising executive.

Barr: (Old English) "a gateway."

Barret: (Teutonic) "mighty as a bear." Also: **Barrett.**

Barris: (Old Welsh) "son of Harry."

Barry: (Celtic) "spear." Also: **Barre, Barrie.** *See also* Baruch, Berry.

Bart, Barth: *see* Bartholomew, Barton.

Bartholomew: (Hebrew) "son of the furrows; a farmer." Biblical: one of the twelve disciples. Also: **Bardo, Bart, Barth, Barthol, Bartholemy, Bartholome (Fr), Barlett, Bartley, Bartolome (Sp), Barton.**

Bartley: (Old English) "Bart's

meadow." *See also* Bartholomew.

Barton: variant of Bartholomew.

Bartram: *see* Bertram.

Baruch: (Hebrew) "blessed." Biblical: disciple of Jeremiah. Also: **Barney, Barrie, Barry.**

Basil: (Greek) "kingly." Saint Basil the Great; Basil Rathbone, actor. Also: **Bas, Basilio (Sp), Baz, Bazyli, Vasilii (Russ).**

Bassett: (Old French) in geology and mining, an outcrop.

Bastian, Bastien: *see* Sebastian.

Bautista: (Spanish) "baptizer; St. John the Baptist."

Baxter: (Teutonic) "the baker."

Bayard: (French) "of the fiery hair." Bayard Taylor, American poet.

Bayley: *see* Bailey.

Beacher: (Old English) "dweller by the beech tree." Also: **Beach.**

Beagan: (Irish Gaelic) "little one."

Beal: (Old French) "handsome one." Also: **Beale.**

Beaman: (Old English) "beekeeper."

Beamer: (Old English) "trumpeter."

Bear: contemporary nickname. Bear Bryant, football coach.

Beattie: (Irish Gaelic) "public victualer."

Beau: (French) "handsome." Also a familiar form of names beginning Beau-. Beau Bridges, actor.
Also: **Bo.**

Beauford, Beaufort: (Old French) "from the beautiful stronghold."

Beaumont: (Old French) "from the beautiful mountain." Beaumont Newhall, historian.

Beauregard: (Old French) "from the fair view site."
Also: **Beau.**

Beck: (Middle English) "a brook."
Also: **Bech, Becker, Beckett.**

Bedwin: (Welsh) "birch tree."

Beecher: see Beacher.

Bela: (Hebrew) "eloquent."

Belden: (Old English) "dweller in the beautiful glen."

Belindo: (Italian) "handsome."

Bellamy: (Old French) "handsome friend."
Also: **Bell.**

Belmont: (Latin) "dweller on the beautiful mountain."
Also: **Belmonte.**

Ben: (Hebrew) "son." Short form of names beginning Ben-. (Chinese) "foundation." See also Benedict, Benjamin.

Benedict: (Latin) "blessed." St. Benedict, founder of the Benedictines.

Also: **Ben, Bendek, Benedic, Benedick, Benedix, Benes, Benito (It/Sp), Bennet, Bennett, Benny, Benoit (Fr).**

Benigno: (Latin) "kind."

Benito: see Benedict. Benito Juarez, president of Mexico.

Benjamin: (Hebrew) "son of my right hand." Biblical: son of Jacob and Rachel.
Also: **Ben, Benson, Benjie, Benjy, Bennie, Benny.**

Bennett: see Benedict. Bennett Cerf, publisher.
Also: **Bennet.**

Benson: see Benjamin.

Bentley: (Old English) "from the bent-grass meadow."

Benton: (Anglo-Saxon) "of the moors."

Berend: (Teutonic) "bear."
Also: **Barend.**

Berenger: "bear spear."

Beresford: (Old English) "from the barley ford."

Berg: (German) "from the mountain." See also Burgess.

Berger: (French) "shepherd." See also Burgess.

Bergin: (Teutonic) "mountain dweller."
Also: **Berg, Bergen.**

Bergstrom: (Swiss) "mountain stream."

Berkeley: (Anglo-Saxon) "from the birch meadow."
Also: **Barclay, Berkley.**

Bern: Scandinavian form of Bernard.
Also: **Berne, Bernie, Bjorn.**

Bernard: (Teutonic) "bear."
Bernard Malamud, author.
Also: **Barnard, Barnet, Barnett,
Barney, Baynard, Bern,
Bernardo (Sp), Bernarr,
Bernhard, Bernie.**

Bernhard: *see* Bernard.

Berry: (English) "berry." Also
a French place name (Berri).
See also Barry.

Bert: (Old English) "bright."
See also Albert, Bertram,
Burton, Egbert, Herbert, etc.

Berthold: (Old German) "brilliant ruler." Bertolt Brecht,
dramatist.

Berton: *see* Burton.

Bertram: (Latin) "bright
raven." Bertrand Russell,
philosopher.
Also: **Bartram, Bert.**

Bertrand: *see* Bertram.

Beryl: (English/Greek) a gem
name.

Bevan: (Celtic) "son of Evan."
Also: **Bevin.**

Beverley: (Anglo-Saxon)
"from the beaver meadow."
Also: **Beverly.**

Bevis: (Old French) "fair
view."

Bickford: (Old English)
"hewer's ford."

Bijan: (Persian) "ancient
hero."

Bill, Billy: *see* William.

Bing: (Old German) "from the
kettle-shaped hollow." Bing
Crosby, actor/singer.

Birch: (Old English) "the
birch tree." Birch Bayh, U.S.
senator.

Also: **Bircher, Birchet.** *See also*
Bedwin.

Birkett: (Middle English)
"dweller at the birch headland."

Birkey: (North English) "from
the birch-tree island."

Birley: (Old English) "cattle
shed on the meadow."

Birney: (Old English) "dweller
on the brook island."

Birtle: (Old English) "from the
bird hill."

Bishop: (Old English) "the
bishop."

Bjorn: (Scandinavian) "bear."
Bjorn Borg, tennis player.

Blackmore: (Teutonic)
"dweller at the black
moor."

Blade: (Old English) "prosperity, glory."

Blagden: (Old English) "from
the dark valley."

Blaine: (Irish Gaelic) "thin,
lean."
Also: **Blane, Blayne.**

Blair: (Celtic) "marshy plain."
Blair Underwood, actor.

Blaise: *see* Blaze. Blaise Pascal, French scientist.

Blake: (Old English) "dark;
dark-complexioned." Blake
Edwards, film director.
Also: **Blakesley.**

Blakeley: (Old English) "from
the black meadow."

Blane: *see* Blaine.

Blanford: (Old English)
"Gray-haired one's river
crossing."

Blayne: *see* Blaine.

Blaze: (Latin) "stammerer." Also: **Blaise, Blase.**

Blessing: (Old English) "consecrated one."

Bliss: (Old English) "joyful one." Bliss Perry, scholar.

Blue: (English) "blue."

Blythe: (Old English) "merry one."

Bo: (Chinese) "the eldest brother; thriving; wealthy." A prefix often combined with another name. Also a Scandinavian nickname. *See also* Beau.

Boaz: (Hebrew) "strength is in the Lord." Biblical: a main character in the Book of Ruth.

Bob, Bobby: *see* Robert.

Boden: (Old French) "herald; messenger." Also: **Bodin.**

Bogart: (Old German) "bow-strong." Bogart Carlaw, advertising executive.

Bolton: (Old English) "manor farm."

Bonar: (Old French) "kind, gentle."

Boniface: (Latin) "doer of good." Saint Boniface. Also: **Bonifacio.**

Booker: "beech tree." Also an occupational name for one who copies books. Booker T. Washington, educator.

Boone: (Old French) "good one." Daniel Boone, frontiersman.

Booth: (Teutonic) "from a market; home-lover." Booth Tarkington, writer.

Borden: (Old English) "he lives near the boar's den." Borden Chase, screenwriter. Also: **Barden.**

Borg: (Norse) "castle dweller."

Boris: (Slavic) "a fighter." Boris Becker, tennis player.

Boston: the name of the city used as a first name.

Boswell: (Old French) "forest town." James Boswell, biographer of Samuel Johnson.

Bosworth: (Old English) "at the cattle enclosure."

Botolf: (Old English) "herald wolf."

Bourne: (Old English) "from the brook."

Boutros: (Arabic) Peter. Boutros Boutros-Ghali, U.N. secretary-general.

Bowen: (Celtic) "the son; descendant of Owen."

Bowie: (Irish Gaelic) "yellow-haired." James Bowie, hero of the Alamo.

Boyce: (Old French) "from the forest."

Boyd: (Celtic) "light-haired." Boyd Matson, television commentator.

Boyne: (Irish Gaelic) "white cow."

Brad: short form of Bradford, Bradley, but also used as an independent name.

Bradburn: (Old English) "broad brook."

Braddock: (English) "from the broad oak."

Braden: (Old English) "from the wide valley."
Also: **Braddon, Braydon.**

Bradford: (Anglo-Saxon) "from the broad ford."
Also: **Brad, Ford.**

Bradley: (Anglo-Saxon) "from the broad meadow."
Also: **Brad.**

Brady: (Irish Gaelic) "spirited one."

Brainard: (Old English) "bold raven."
Also: **Brainerd.**

Bram: *see* Abraham, Bramwell. Bram Stoker, author of *Dracula.*

Bramwell: (Old English) "of Abraham's well."
Also: **Bram.**

Branch: (English) "bow; a name referring to the Day of Branches, Palm Sunday." Branch Rickey, baseball general manager.

Brand: (Old English) "firebrand." Brandel Chamblee, golfer.
Also: **Brander, Brandt, Brant.**

Brandon: *see* Brendan.

Branford: a variant of the English surname Bramford. Branford Marsalis, jazz musician.

Brant: variant of Brand.

Brawley: (Old English) "from the hill-slope meadow."

Braxton: (Old English) "one who lives at the boundary."

Braxton Bragg, Confederate general.

Brendan: (Celtic) "from the fiery hill." Brendan Behan, Irish writer.
Also: **Brandon, Brannon, Brendon, Brennan.**

Brent: (Teutonic) "steep hill."
Also: **Brendt.**

Brett: (French) "a native of Brittany." Bret Harte, writer (1836–1902).
Also: **Bret, Britt.**

Brewster: (Old English) "brewer." Brewster Shaw, U.S. astronaut.

Brian: (Celtic) "strong; powerful." Brian Boru, king of Ireland.
Also: **Briant, Brion, Bryan, Bryant.**

Brice: (Celtic) "ambitious; alert."
Also: **Bryce.**

Brick: (English) "bridge."

Bridger: (Old English) "bridge builder." James Bridger, mountain man.

Brier: (Old English) "the briers."

Brigham: (Anglo-Saxon) "a dweller by the bridge."

Brittan: (Latin) "from Brittany." Britt Hume, TV correspondent.
Also: **Briton, Britt, Brittain.**

Brock: (Celtic) "badger." Brock Peters, actor.
Also: **Brocker.**

Brockley: (Old English) "from the badger meadow."

Broderick: *see* Roderick.

Brodie: (Irish Gaelic) "a ditch."
Also: **Brody.**

Bromley: (Old English) "a dweller in the meadow."
Also: **Bromlea, Bromleigh.**

Bronson: (Old English) "son of the brown one." Bronson Pinchot, actor.

Brook: (Middle English) "brook or stream."
Also: **Brooker.**

Brooklyn: Brooklyn Demme, son of Jonathan Demme, film director.

Brooks: (Middle English) variant of Brook. Brooks Atkinson, drama critic.
Also: **Brookes.**

Brougher: (Old English) "fortress resident."

Broughton: (Old English) "from the fortress town."

Brown: (Middle English) "dark, reddish complexion."

Bruce: Scottish surname. Robert the Bruce, king of Scotland. Bruce Catton, writer.

Bruno: (Teutonic) "brown." Bruno Bettelheim, psychologist and educator.

Bryan, Bryant: *see* Brian. Bryant Gumbel, broadcaster.

Bryce: *see* Brice.

Bryn: (Welsh) "hill."
Also: **Brynn.**

Buck: (Old English) "buck deer." Buck Henry, actor/writer.
Also: **Bucky.**

Buckley: (Old English) "dweller at the buck deer meadow."

Bud/Budd: (Gaelic) "messenger." Buddy Holly, rock musician (1936–1959).

Bundy: (Old English) "free man."

Burbank: (Old English) "dweller on the castle-hill slope."

Burch: (Middle English) "birch tree."
Also: **Burcher.**

Burchard: (Old English) "strong as a castle."

Burdett: (Old French) "little shield."
Also: **Burditt.**

Burdon: (Old English) "dweller at the castle hill."

Burford: (Old English) "dweller at the castle ford."

Burgess: (Teutonic) "a townsman." Burgess Meredith, actor.
Also: **Berg, Berger, Bergess, Burg.**

Burke: (Teutonic) "from the stronghold; castle."
Also: **Berk, Birk, Bourke, Burk.**

Burl: (Old English) "cupbearer." Burl Ives, folk singer.

Burley: (Old English) "dweller at the castle meadow."
Also: **Burleigh.**

Burne: (Old English) "brook."

Burnell: (Old English) "little brown-haired one."

Burnett: (Middle English) "little brown-complected one."

Burney: (Old English) "dweller at the brook island."

Burr: (Old Norse) "youth."

Burrell: (Old French) "reddish-brown complexion."

Burroughs: (Teutonic) "dweller at a stronghold." John Burroughs, naturalist.
Also: **Burrough, Burrows.**

Burt: *see* Burton.

Burton: (Anglo-Saxon) "fortified enclosure." Burton Lane, Broadway and film composer.
Also: **Bert, Berton, Burt.**

Busby: (Scotch-Norse) "dweller at the village in the thicket."

Byford: (Old English) "dweller at the river crossing."

Byram: (Old English) "dweller at the cattle-shed place."

Byrd: (Old English) "birdlike."

Byron: (French) "from the cottage; the bear." Byron Nelson, golfer.

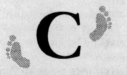

Cable: (French) "rope." Cab Calloway, singer.
Also: **Cabell.**

Cadby: (Old Norse-English) "warrior's settlement."

Caddock: (Old Welsh) "battle keenness."

Cadell: (Old Welsh) "battle spirit."
Also: **Cadel.**

Cadman: (Celtic) "brave warrior."

Cadmus: (Greek) "man from the East." Mythology: Cadmus was the founder of Thebes.

Cador: (Welsh) "mighty; shield."

Caesar: (Latin) "born with long hair; leader."
Also: **Cesar (Sp).**

Cain: (Hebrew) "possession or possessed." Biblical: murderer of his brother Abel.

Caius: *see* Gaius.

Cal: *see* Caleb, Calvin.

Calder: (Celtic) "from the river of stones."

Caldwell: (Old English) "cold spring."
Also: **Colwell.**

Caleb: (Hebrew) "bold; impetuous." Cale Yarborough, race car driver. Biblical: one of the spies sent by Moses to Canaan.
Also: **Cal.**

Caley: (Irish Gaelic) "thin, slender."

Calhoun: (Irish Gaelic) "from the narrow forest."

Callan: (Irish) "battle-mighty."
Also: **Callen.**

Callisto: (Greek) "beautiful."
Also: **Calisto, Calixto.**

Callum: (Celtic) "dove."

Calvert: (Old English) "herdsman."

Calvin: (Latin) "bald." Calvin Trillin, journalist and author.
Also: **Cal, Calvert.**

Camden: (Anglo-Gaelic) "from the winding valley."

Cameron: (Celtic) "bent nose." Cameron Crowe, film director.
Also: **Cam.**

Camilo: (Spanish) "freeborn." Camilo Pessanha, poet.
Also: **Camillo.**

Campbell: (French) "from a bright field."
Also: **Cam.**

Canute: (Old Norse) "knot." Canute, king of England, Denmark, and Norway.

Canyon: a contemporary name. Canyon Ceman, volleyball player.

Carew: (Celtic) "from this fortress."
Also: **Carr.**

Carey: see Charles.

Carl: variant of Charles. Carl Sandburg, poet. See also Karl.

Carleton: (Old English) "farmer's settlement." Carlton Fisk, baseball player.
Also: **Carlton.** See also Charlton.

Carlin: (Irish Gaelic) "little champion."
Also: **Carlan.**

Carlisle: (Latin) "from a walled city; island."
Also: **Carlyle.**

Carlos: see Charles.

Carlton: see Carleton.

Carmelo: (Hebrew) "God's fruitful field." Biblical: Mount Carmel.
Also: **Carmelito.**

Carmichael: (Scotch Gaelic) "friend of St. Michael."

Carmine: (Italian) "vineyard."

Carney: (Irish Gaelic) "victorious." Carney Lansford, baseball player.
Also: **Carny.**

Carollan: (Irish Gaelic) "little champion."

Carr: (Old Norse) "dweller at a marsh." See also Carew.

Carrick: (Irish Gaelic) "rocky headland."

Carroll: (Irish Gaelic) "champion." Carroll O'Connor, actor.
Also: **Carol, Carrol.**

Carson: (Scottish) "dweller by the marshes."

Carswell: (Old English) "dweller at the watercress spring."

Carter: (Anglo-Saxon) "cartmaker." Carter Braxton, member of Continental Congress.

Cartland: (Scotch-English) "land between the streams."

Carvell: (Old French) "spearman's estate."

Carver: (Anglo-Saxon) "one who carves."

Carvey: (Irish Gaelic) "athlete."

Cary: (Old Welsh) "dweller at the castles." Cary Grant, actor.

Casey: (Celtic) "brave." Casey

Stengel, baseball player, manager.

Cash: (Latin) "vain one."

Cashel: an Irish place name.

Casimir: (Slavic) "proclamation of peace." Casimir the Great, king of Poland.
Also: **Casper, Cass, Kasimir, Kazimir.**

Caspar, Casper: see Casimir, Jasper.

Cassidy: (Irish Gaelic) "curly-haired."

Cassius: (Latin) "vain." Cassius Clay (later Muhammad Ali), heavyweight champion.
Also: **Cass, Casseus.**

Castor: (Greek) "beaver."

Cathal: (Irish) "battle-mighty."
Also: **Cahal, Cahir.**

Cathmor: (Irish Gaelic) "great warrior."

Cato: (Latin) "wise one."

Cavanaugh: (Irish Gaelic) "handsome."
Also: **Cavan, Kavan.**

Cavell: (Old French) "little active one."

Cawley: (Scotch-Norse) "ancestral relic."

Cecil: (Latin) "blind." Cecil B. DeMille, film director; Cecil Beaton, photographer.
Also: **Cecilio (Sp).**

Cedar: (English) "cedar tree." Cedar Walton, jazz artist.

Cedric: (Celtic) "chieftain." Cedric Dempsey, executive director, NCAA.
Also: **Cedrick, Cedro.**

Cerwin: (Welsh) "fair love."
Also: **Cerwyn.**

Cesar: see Caesar. Cesar Chavez, labor leader.
Also: **Cesare.**

Cezanne: a contemporary name inspired by the French Impressionist painter Paul Cezanne.

Chad: (Old English) "war-like."

Chadwick: (Celtic) "defender."
Also: **Chad.**

Chaim: (Hebrew) "life." Chaim Soutine, artist.
Also: **Hy, Hyam, Hyman, Mannie, Manny.**

Chalmer: (Teutonic) "king of the household."
Also: **Chalmers.**

Chance: (Middle English) "good fortune." Chance Gardiner, feature character in Jerzy Kosinski's novel *Being There.*

Chancelor: see Chauncey.

Chandler: (French) "candlemaker."
Also: **Chan.**

Chaney: see Cheney.

Chang: (Chinese) "prosperous." Traditionally combined with a second name.

Channing: (Anglo-Saxon) "a regent; knowing."

Chapin: (French) "a man of God."
Also: **Chapen, Chapland, Chaplin.**

Chappell: (English) "dweller near a chapel."
Also: **Chapel, Chappell.**

Charles: (Teutonic) "man." Charles I, king of England.
Also: **Carl, Carlo, Carlos, Carol, Carrol, Charley, Charlie, Chas, Chuck, Karl, Karol (Pol).** *See also* Karl.

Charlton: (Anglo-Saxon) "of Charles' farm." Charlton Heston, actor.
Also: **Carleton, Carlton, Charleton.**

Chase: (Old French) "hunter."
Also: **Chasen.**

Chatham: (Old English) "soldier's land."

Chauncey: (French) "official record keeper."
Also: **Chancelor, Chancellor.**

Chayton: (American Indian— Sioux) "falcon."

Chen: (Chinese) "treasure; star; morning." Traditionally combined with a second name. Chen Kaige, film director.

Cheney: (Old French) "dweller at the oak forest."
Also: **Chaney, Chesney.**

Cherokee: (American Indian) "people of a different speech."

Chester: (Latin) "of the fortified camp." Chester Alan Arthur, 21st U.S. President.
Also: **Cheston, Chet.**

Chet: *see* Chester. Chet Huntley, newscaster.

Chetwin: (Old English) "from the cottage on the winding path."

Chevy: (French) "horseman; knight." A short form of Chevalier. Chevy Chase, actor, comedian.
Also: **Cheval.**

Cheyenne: (French/American Indian) name of an Algonquian tribe of the Great Plains.

Chilton: (Anglo-Saxon) "from the farm by the spring."

Chisholm: (Teutonic) "dweller on the gravel island."

Christian: (Latin) "a Christian." Christiaan Barnard, surgeon; performed first human heart transplant.
Also: **Chretien, Chris, Christen, Christos (Gr), Kit, Kristian, Kristin.**

Christopher: (Greek) "Christ-bearer." St. Christopher, patron saint of travelers.
Also: **Chris, Christoph, Christophe (Fr), Christy, Cristoval (Sp), Kester, Kit, Kris, Kriss.**

Chuan: (Chinese) "to pass down; river."

Chuck: *see* Charles.

Chuma: (Swahili) "strong."

Churchill: (Old English) "dweller at the church hill."

Cian: (Irish Gaelic) "ancient one."

Cicero: (Latin) "chickpea." Cicero, Roman statesman.

Ciprian: *see* Cyprian.

Clair, Claire: (Latin) "famous one." Claire Chennault, U.S. Air Force general. *See also* Clarence.

Clancy: (Irish) "redheaded fighter."
Also: **Clancey.**

Clarence: (Latin) "bright, shining, gentle."

Clark: (Latin) "scholarly; wise."
Also: **Clarke.**

Claud, Claude: (Latin) "lame." Claude Debussy, French composer.
Also: **Claudio (Sp), Claudy.**

Claus: see Nicholas.

Clay: see Clayton.

Clayton: (Anglo-Saxon) "mortal man."
Also: **Clay, Clayborn, Clayborne.**

Cleary: (Irish Gaelic) "scholar."

Cleavon: (Old English) "cliff." Cleavon Little, actor.
Also: **Cleavant.**

Clem: see Clement.

Clement: (Latin) "mild; kind; merciful." Saint Clement of Alexandria; Saint Clement I.
Also: **Clem, Clemence, Clemens, Clemente.**

Cleve: see Clive.

Cleveland: (Old English) "from the cliff island." Cleveland Abbe, astronomer.
Also: **Cleve.**

Cliff: (Anglo-Saxon) "a headland."
Also: **Cliffe.** See also Clifford, Clifton.

Clifford: (Anglo-Saxon) "from the ford near the cliff." Clifford Odets, playwright.
Also: **Cliff.**

Clifton: (Anglo-Saxon) "from the farm at the cliff."

Clinton: (Anglo-Saxon) "from the headland farm." Clint Eastwood, actor, filmmaker. Clint Black, country singer.

Clive: (Anglo-Saxon) "cliff." Clive Barnes, journalist, critic.
Also: **Cleve, Clyve.**

Clovis: see Lewis. Clovis, king of the Franks.

Cluny: (Irish Gaelic) "from the meadow."

Clyde: (Celtic) the Scottish river and surname. Clyde Fitch, dramatist.

Clymer: signer of the Declaration of Independence.

Cobb: a diminutive of Jacob.

Cody: (Irish/English) "helpful."
Also: **Codey, Codie, Kody.**

Colan: see Colin.

Colbert: (Old English) "brilliant seafarer."

Colby: (Old English) "from the dark farm."

Cole: a short form of Nicholas and other names beginning Col-. Cole Porter, lyricist, composer. See also Clarence, Coleman, Colin.

Coleman: (Celtic) "dove keeper." Coleman Hawkins, jazz saxophonist (1901–1969).
Also: **Col, Cole, Colman.**

Colin: (Celtic) "strong; young and virile." General Colin Powell, chairman of the Joint Chiefs of Staff (ret.)

Also: **Colan, Cole, Collin.** *See also* Nicholas.

Colley: *see* Nicholas.

Collier: (Old English) "miner."

Colm: (Irish) "dove." Colm Meaney, actor. St. Columba.
Also: **Colum.**

Colt: (English) "young horse; frisky."

Colter: (Old English) "colt herder."
Also: **Coulter.**

Colton: (Old English) "from the dark estate."

Colum: *see* Colm.

Colver: *see* Culver.

Comfort: Puritan name used for both sexes.

Conal: (Celtic) "high and mighty."
Also: **Con, Conall, Conana, Conant, Conn, Connel, Kynan, Quinn.**

Conan: (Celtic) "intelligence." Conan O'Brien, talk show host. *See also* Conal.

Conant: *see* Conal.

Conlan: (Irish Gaelic) "hero." Conley Verdun, basketball player.
Also: **Conlon.**

Connie: contemporary nickname and short form of names beginning Con-. Connie (Cornelius) Mack, baseball player, manager.

Connor: (Irish) "hound-lover."
Also: **Conner, Connie, Conor.**

Conrad: (Teutonic) "brave counsel." Conrad Aiken, poet.

Also: **Con, Connie, Curt, Konrad, Kurt.**

Conroy: (Celtic) "wise."
Also: **Connie.**

Constantine: (Latin) "unwavering; firm." Constantine the Great, emperor of Rome; Constantin Costa-Gavras, film director; Constantin Brancusi, sculptor.
Also: **Connie, Constancio (Sp), Constant, Constantino.**

Conway: (Celtic) "a man of the great plains." Conway Twitty, country singer.
Also: **Connie.**

Cooper: (Old English) "barrel maker."

Corbett: (Old French) "raven."
Also: **Corbet.**

Corbin: (Latin) "the raven." Corbin Bernsen, actor.
Also: **Corby, Corwin.**

Corcoran: (Irish Gaelic) "reddish complexion."

Cordell: (French) "binding cord; rope."
Also: **Cord.**

Corey: (Celtic) "ravine dweller."
Also: **Corley, Cory, Korey.**

Cormac: (Irish Gaelic) "charioteer; son of the raven." Cormac McCarthy, novelist.
Also: **Cormack.**

Cormick: a form of Cormac.

Cornelius: (Latin) "battle horn."
Also: **Connie, Cornel, Cornell, Neal, Neil, Nelson.**

Cornell: (Old French) "horn-colored hair." Cornel Wilde,

actor; Cornell Capa, photographer.
Also: **Kornel.** *See also* Cornelius.

Cort: *see* Courtenay.

Cortez: a Spanish surname. Cortez Kennedy, football player.

Corwin: *see* Corbin.

Corydon: (Greek) "crested one."

Cosmo: (Greek) "universe; in good order."

Cotton: (Anglo-Saxon) "at the cottages." Colonial figure Cotton Mather.

Courtenay: a French place name.
Also: **Cort, Court, Courtland, Courtney.**

Covell: (Old English) "dweller at the cave slope."

Cowan: (Irish Gaelic) "hillside valley."

Coyle: (Irish Gaelic) "battle follower."

Craddock: (Old Welsh) "abounding in love."

Craig: (Celtic) "of the crag; stony hill."
Also: **Cragg.**

Crandall: (Old English) "of the valley of the cranes; caretaker of the cranes."

Cranley: (Old English) "from the crane meadow."

Cranston: (Old English) "from the crane town."

Crawford: (Old English) "of the crow's crossing."

Creighton: (Middle English) "dweller at the creek town."

Creighton Abrams, U.S. general.

Crispin: (Latin) "curly-haired." Crispin Glover, actor.
Also: **Crispen.**

Crockett: (English) "crooked." Crockett Johnson, cartoonist, illustrator.

Cromwell: (Old English) "dweller at the winding stream."

Crosby: (Anglo-Saxon) "near the crossroad."

Crosley: (Old English) "from the cross meadow."

Cruz: (Spanish) "cross."

Cuba: a contemporary use of the place name. Cuba Gooding, actor.

Culbert: (Teutonic) "noted and bright."
Also: **Colbert, Cuthbert.**

Cullen: (Irish Gaelic) "handsome one."

Culley: (Irish Gaelic) "at the woodland."

Culver: (Anglo-Saxon) "gentle; peaceful; dove."
Also: **Colver.**

Curran: (origin uncertain) "heroic; resolute."
Also: **Curry.**

Curt: *see* Conrad, Curtis.

Curtis: (French) "courteous."
Also: **Curt, Curtiss, Kurt.**

Cuthbert: *see* Culbert.

Cutler: (Old English) "the knife maker."

Cy: short form of names beginning Cy-. Cy Coleman, songwriter.

Cynan: (Welsh) "chief, preeminent."
Also: **Cynin, Cynon.**

Cynric: (Old English) "powerful and royal."

Cyprian: (Greek) "man from Cyprus." Saint Cyprian; Cyprian Kamil Norwid, Polish poet.

Cyrano: (Greek) "from Cyrene." Cyrano de Bergerac, hero of the romantic play of that name.

Cyril: (Greek) "lord." St. Cyril of Alexandria.
Also: **Cirilo (Sp), Cyriel.**

Cyrus: (Persian) "throne." Cyrus the Great, king of Persia; Cyrus Adler, American educator. Biblical: founder of the Persian Empire.
Also: **Cy, Russ.**

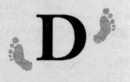

Dabney: surname derived from the French place name Saint-Aubin-d'Aubigne. Dabney Coleman, actor.

Dacey: (Irish Gaelic) "Southerner."
Also: **Dacy.**

Dag: (Old Norse) "day or brightness." Dag Hammarskjöld, U.N. secretary-general.

Dagan: (East Semitic) "the earth; little fish." In Babylonian mythology, the god of the earth and grain.

Dagwood: (Old English) "bright one's forest."

Dakota: (American Indian—Sioux) "alliance of friends."

Dalbert: (Old English) "proud, brilliant one."

Dale: (Teutonic) "valley dweller." Dale Carnegie, teacher of public speaking.
Also: **Dalton.**

Dallan: Dallan Forgaill, 7th-century Irish poet.

Dallas: (Anglo-Saxon) "dweller in the dale."
Also: **Dal.**

Dalton: (Old English) "from the valley town." Dalton Trumbo, blacklisted screenwriter. *See also* Dale.

Daly: (Irish Gaelic) "counselor."

Dalziel: (Scotch Gaelic) "from the little field."

Damian, Damien: *see* Damon. Damian, a patron saint of physicians.

Damon: (Greek) "tame; domesticated." Damon Runyon, writer.
Also: **Daimon, Damian.**

Dana, Dane: (Scandinavian) "a Dane." Dana Andrews, actor.
Also: **Danek.**

Danby: (Old Norse) "from the Dane's settlement." *See also* Denby.

Daniel: (Hebrew) "God is judge." Biblical: the Book of

Daniel. Daniel Webster, American statesman.
Also: **Dan, Daniell, Danilo, Danny, Darnell.**

Danilo: Spanish form of Daniel. Danilo Perez, jazz artist.

Dante: (Italian) "lasting." Dante Alighieri, poet.

Darby: (Irish Gaelic) "free man." Darby Hinton, actor.

Darcy: (French) "from the stronghold."
Also: **D'Arcy.**

Darius: (Persian) "a man of wealth." Biblical: the name of three Persian emperors. Darius Rucker, rock musician, singer.
Also: **Darian, Darren, Derian.**

Darrell: (Anglo-Saxon) "beloved."
Also: **Darren, Darryl, Daryl.**

Darren: diminutive of Darius, Darrell, Dorian, etc., but also used as an independent name.

Darton: (Old English) "deer park."

Darwin: (English) "dweller near clear water." Darwin Cooke, basketball coach.

Daryl: *see* Darrell.

Dashiell: Dashiell Hammett, writer.
Also: **Dash.**

David: (Hebrew) "beloved." Biblical: slayer of Goliath and king of Israel. St. David, patron saint of Wales.
Also: **Dave, Davie, Davis, Davy, Davyn, Dewey.**

Davin: (Scandinavian) "the bright man; bright Finn."

Davis: a form of David. Davis Love III, golfer.
Also: **Davidson, Dawson.**

Deacon, Deakin: a form of David; "deacon or minister." Deacon Jones, football player.
Also: **Deke.**

Dean: (Anglo-Saxon) "valley." Dean Acheson, U.S. secretary of state.
Also: **Deane.**

DeAndre: a contemporary name.

Dearborn: (Anglo-Saxon) "beloved baby; child."

Dedrick: (Old German) "ruler of the people."

Deems: (Old English) "son of the judge."

Dekker: a form of Derek.

Del, Dell: short forms of any name beginning Del-.

Delano: (Old French) "from the place of the nut trees." Franklin Delano Roosevelt, 32nd U.S. President.
Also: **Del, Delaney.**

Delbert: *see* Albert.

Delling: (Old Norse) "very shining one."
Also: **Del.**

Delmar: (Latin) "of the sea." Delmer Daves, film director (1904–1977).
Also: **Del, Delmer.**

Delwyn: (Old English) "proud friend."

Demas: (Greek) "proud one."

Demetrius: (Greek) "lover of the earth." Biblical: king of

Syria. Demetrius Porter, basketball player.
Also: **Demetrio (Sp), Demmy, Dimitri (Russ), Dmitri.**

Demos: (Greek) "the people."

Dempsey: (Irish Gaelic) "proud one." *See also* Dempster.

Dempster: (Old English) "a judge; wise."
Also: **Dempsey, Dempstor.**

Denby: (Scandinavian) "from the Danish settlement; loyal Dane."
Also: **Danby.**

Denholm: (Scottish) "valley; dry land in a fen." Denholm Elliott, actor.
Also: **Den.**

Denis: *see* Dennis.

Denley: (Old English) "dweller in the valley meadow."

Denman: (Old English) "valley resident."

Dennis: (Greek) "lover of fine wines; follower of Dionysius." St. Denis, patron saint of France.
Also: **Denis, Dennie, Dennison, Denny, Deny, Denys (Fr), Denzil, Dion.**

Dennison: *see* Dennis.

Denny: familiar form of names beginning Den-.

Denton: (Old English) "from the valley estate." Cy (Denton True) Young, baseball pitcher.

Denver: (Old English) "dweller at the valley edge."

Denys: *see* Dennis.

Denzel: Denzel Washington, actor.
Also: **Denzil.** *See also* Dennis.

Derek, Derk, Derrick: Derek Walcott, Nobel prize–winning poet. *See also* Theodoric.

Dermot: *see* Kermit.

Derward: (Old English) "deer warden."

Derwin: (Old English) "beloved friend."

Desmond: (Celtic) "worldly; sophisticated." Bishop Desmond Tutu, winner of the Nobel Peace Prize.
Also: **Desi, Dez.**

Deverell: (Old Welsh-English) "from the riverbank."

Devin: *see* Devon.

Devlin: (Irish Gaelic) "fierce valor."

Devon: an English place name.
Also: **Devin.**

Dewey: *see* David.

De Witt: (Old Flemish) "blond one."

Dexter: (Latin) "right-handed; dexterous." Dexter Gordon, jazz artist.

Diamond: (Old English) "bright protector."

Dick: *see* Richard.

Didier: (French) "beloved." Didier Pitre, hockey player.

Diego: Spanish form of Diego Rivera, Mexican painter.

Digby: (Old Norse) "from the dike settlement."

Dillard: from the English surname Dill. Dillard Pruitt, golfer.

Dillon: (Celtic) "faithful."

Dilwin: a Welsh place name. Also: **Dilwyn.**

Dimitri: (Russian) "follower of Demeter, the Greek goddess of agriculture." Also a saint's name.
Also: **Dimitrios (Gr).**

Dion: a form of Dennis. Deion Sanders, athlete.
Also: **Deion.**

Dirk: a Dutch form of Derrick. Dirk Bogarde, actor.

Dixon: see Benedict.

Doane: (Celtic) "dweller of the sand dune."

Dodge: (English) a pet form of Roger.

Dolan: (Irish Gaelic) "blackhaired."

Dolph: see Adolfo, Rudolph. Dolph Lundgren, actor.

Dominic: (Latin) "the Lord's." St. Dominic. Dominique Wilkins, basketball player.
Also: **Dom, Domenico, Dominick (Pol), Dominico, Dominy, Nic, Nick, Nicky.**

Don: short form of names beginning Don-.

Donald: (Celtic) "ruler of the world." Donald Sutherland, actor.
Also: **Don, Donal, Donaldo (Sp), Donall, Donnell, Donnie, Donny.**

Donato: (Latin) "a gift."

Donegal: (Celtic) "dweller at the foreigner's stronghold." Donegal, the northernmost county of Ireland.

Donovan: (Celtic) "brown one." Donovan Leitch, singer.

Dooley: (Irish Gaelic) "dark hero."

Doran: (Greek) "the stranger."
Also: **Dorran.**

Dorian: (Greek) "from Doris." Dorian Gray, of the Oscar Wilde novel and later film. Dorian Harewood, actor.
Also: **Darren, Dore, Dorey, Dory.** See also Isidore.

Dory: (French) "goldenhaired."
Also: **Dore.**

Douglas: (Celtic) "from the black stream."
Also: **Doug, Dougal.**

Dover: (English) "from Dover." Dover Wilson, British scholar.

Dow: (Irish Gaelic) "blackhaired."

Doyle: (Celtic) "the dark stranger; newcomer."

Drake: (Middle English) "owner of the Dragon Inn sign."

Drew: a form of Andrew.
Also: **Dru, Drue.**

Driscoll: (Celtic) "the speaker or interpreter."

Druce: (Celtic) "wise man; capable and adept."

Drury: (Old French) "sweetheart."

Duane: (Celtic) "son of the little dark one."
Also: **Dwane, Dwayne.**

Duarte: Portuguese form of Edward.

Dudley: (Anglo-Saxon) "a place." Dudley Moore, British actor.
Also: **Lee.**

Duff: (Irish Gaelic) "dark-complexioned one."

Dugan: (Irish Gaelic) "dark-complexioned."

Duke: (Latin) "leader." Duke Kahanamoku, Olympic swimmer.

Duncan: (Celtic) "warrior of dark skin." Duncan Phyfe, cabinetmaker.
Also: **Dunc.**

Dunley: (Old English) "from the hill meadow."

Dunmore: (Scotch Gaelic) "great hill fortress."

Dunn: (Old English) "dark-complexioned one."

Dunstan: (Anglo-Saxon) "from the brown stone hill." Saint Dunstan.

Dunton: (Old English) "of the farm over the hill."

Durand: (Latin) "enduring."
Also: **Duran, Durant.**

Durward: (Anglo-Saxon) "the doorkeeper."
Also: **Derwood, Durware, Durwood.**

Durwin: (Anglo-Saxon) "dear friend."
Also: **Durwyn.**

Dustin: (Teutonic) "strong-hearted leader." Dustin Hoffman, actor.

Dutch: (German) "the German."

Dwayne: see Duane.

Dwight: (Teutonic) "light." Dwight Eisenhower, 34th U.S. President.

Dylan: (Old Welsh) "from the sea." Dylan Thomas, poet.
Also: **Dyllon.** See also Dillon.

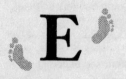

E

Eachan: (Irish Gaelic) "little horse."
Also: **Eachann.**

Eamon: (Irish) "fortunate; rich protector." Eamon de Valera, Irish statesman.
Also: **Eames.**

Earl: (Anglo-Saxon) "nobleman; chief." Earl Warren, 14th chief justice of the Supreme Court.
Also: **Earle, Early, Erle, Errol.**

Earnest: see Ernest.

Eaton: (Anglo-Saxon) "of the river; riverside."

Eben: (Hebrew) "stone." Eben Tourjee, founder of the New England Conservatory of Music.
Also: **Eban.**

Ebenezer: (Hebrew) "stone of help." Ebenezer Zane, Revolutionary War figure.
Also: **Eb, Eben.**

Eberhart: *see* Everard.

Ebner: (German) "dweller in the lowlands."

Edan: (Celtic) "flame."

Edbert: (Old English) "prosperous; brilliant."

Edel: (Old German) "noble one."

Edelmar: (Old English) "noble; famous."

Eden: (Hebrew) "place of delight and pleasure." Eden Phillpotts, British novelist.

Edgar: (Anglo-Saxon) "lucky spear; fortunate warrior." Edgar the Peaceful, king of England; Edgar Allan Poe, writer.
Also: **Ed, Eddie.**

Edison: (Old English) "Edward's son."
Also: **Edson.**

Edlin: *see* Edwin.

Edmund: (Anglo-Saxon) "fortunate; rich protector." Sir Edmund Hillary, explorer.
Also: **Ed, Eddie, Edmon, Edmond, Edmundo (Sp).**

Edolf: (Old English) "prosperous wolf."

Edred: (Old English) "fortunate counsel."

Edric: (Anglo-Saxon) "rich ruler."
Also: **Edrick.**

Edsel: (Anglo-Saxon) "profound; deep thinker."

Edson: *see* Edison.

Edwald: (Old English) "prosperous ruler."

Edward: (Anglo-Saxon) "prosperous guardian." Edward the Confessor, king of England.
Also: **Duarte, Ed, Eddie, Eddy, Eduard (Fr), Eduardo (Sp), Ted, Teddy.**

Edwin: (Anglo-Saxon) "wealthy friend." Edwin Land, inventor of the Polaroid Land camera.
Also: **Ed, Eddie, Eddy, Edlin.**

Efrem: *see* Ephraim.

Egan: (Teutonic) "formidable."
Also: **Egon.**

Egbert: (Anglo-Saxon) "bright and shining sword."
Also: **Bert, Bertie.**

Ehren: (Old German) "honorable one."

Einar: (Old Norse) "warrior leader."

Elbert: *see* Albert.

Elder: (English) "dweller near the elder tree."

Eldon: (Teutonic) "respected; older." Elden Campbell, basketball player.
Also: **El, Elden.**

Eldridge: (Teutonic) "wise adviser." Eldrick (Tiger) Woods, golfer.
Also: **Eldred, Eldrid.**

Eldwin: (Anglo-Saxon) "wise friend; adviser."
Also: **Eldwen.**

Eleazar: (Hebrew) "helped by God." Biblical: the son of Aaron. Eleazar Wheelock, Dartmouth College founder.
Also: **Eliezer, Lazar, Lazarus.**

Eleph: (Hebrew) "strong as an ox."

Elgin: (English) "noble." Elgin Baylor, basketball player.

Eli: (Hebrew) "the highest." Biblical: the highest priest of Israel, mentor of Samuel. Eli Whitney, inventor of the cotton gin.
Also: **Elia, Ely.**

Elias: (Hebrew) a form of Elijah; "my God is Jehovah." Elia Kazan, film director.
Also: **Ellis.**

Elihu: (Hebrew) "God, the Lord." Elihu Burritt, 19th-century peace activist. *See also* Elias.

Elijah: (Hebrew) "the Lord is God." Biblical: Elijah the prophet. Elijah Wood, actor.

Elio: (Spanish) "the sun."
Also: **Helio.**

Eliot: (Hebrew) "the Lord is God."
Also: **Elihu, Elijah, Eliot, Elliot, Ellis.**

Elisha: (Hebrew) "God, my salvation." Biblical: the successor of Elijah.

Elizer: Elie Wiesel, winner of the Nobel Peace Prize.

Ellard: (Teutonic) "nobly brave."

Ellery: (Teutonic) "of the alder trees." Ellery Queen, famous fictional character and pseudonym.
Also: **Elery.**

Elliot: *see* Eliot.

Ellis: a form of Elias. Ellis Marsalis, music educator.

Ellison: (Hebrew) "son of Elias." Ellison Onizuka, first Asian-American in space.
Also: **Elison.**

Ellsworth: (Anglo-Saxon) "lover of the earth; farmer." Ellsworth Kelly, artist.
Also: **Elsworth.**

Elmer: (Anglo-Saxon) "noble; famous."
Also: **Aylmer.**

Elmo: (Greek) "friendly." Elmo R. Zumwalt, Jr., U.S. admiral.

Elmore: (Old English) "dweller at the elm-tree moor." Elmore Leonard, author.

Elroy: (Latin) "royal."
Also: **Leroy, Roy.**

Elsdon: (Old English) "noble one's hill."

Elston: (Old English) "noble one's town."

Elsworth: (Old English) "noble one's estate." *See also* Ellsworth.

Elton: (Anglo-Saxon) "from the old farm; village." Elton John, pop singer, songwriter.

Elvin: *see* Alvin. Elvin Hayes, basketball player.

Elvis: (Old Norse) "all-wise."
Also: **Alvis.**

Elvy: (Old English) "elfin warrior."

Elwell: (Old English) "from the old spring."

Elwin: (Anglo-Saxon) "a friend of elves."
Also: **Elwyn, Winn, Wynn.**

Elwood: (Old English) "from the old forest." Ellwood

Kieser, Roman Catholic priest and film producer.

Emanuel: *see* Emmanuel.

Emerson: (Old English) "son of Emory." Also the American poet and philosopher Ralph Waldo Emerson. Emerson Fittipaldi, race car driver.

Emery: *see* Emory.

Emil: (Teutonic) "industrious." Also: **Emile (Fr), Emilio, Emlyn.**

Emilio: Spanish form of Emil. Emilio Estevez, actor; Emiliano Zapata, revolutionary hero of Mexico.

Emlyn: a Welsh place name. Emlyn Williams, Welsh playwright, actor; Emlyn Aubrey, golfer.

Emmanuel: (Hebrew) "God is with us." Emanuel Swedenborg, Swedish scientist, mystic. Also: **Emanuel, Immanuel, Manuel, Manny.**

Emmet: (Anglo-Saxon) "ant; industrious." Emmitt Smith, football player. Also: **Em, Emmett.**

Emory: (Teutonic) "work leader; ambitious." Also: **Emery.**

Emrys: a Welsh form of Ambrose.

Ennis: (Irish Gaelic) "one choice." An Irish place name.

Enoch: (Hebrew) "devoted." Biblical: the father of Methuselah.

Enos: (Hebrew) "mortal." Bib-lical: Enos, the son of Seth. Enos Barton, manufacturer.

Enrico: *see* Henry. Enrico Caruso, opera singer.

Enrique: *see* Henry.

Enzo: Italian form of Henry.

Ephraim: (Hebrew) "fruitful." Biblical: son of Joseph. Also: **Efrain (Sp), Efrem.**

Erasmus: (Greek) "kindly." Also: **Erasmo (Sp).**

Erastus: (Greek) "beloved." Also: **Rasmus, Rastus.**

Erhard: (Teutonic) "honor." Also: **Erhardt, Erhart.**

Eric: (Teutonic) "kingly." Eric Rohmer, French filmmaker. Also: **Erich (Ger), Erick, Erik, Eriq (Fr), Rick, Ricky.**

Erland: (Teutonic) "noble eagle."

Erle: *see* Earl. Erle Stanley Gardner, author.

Erling: (Old English) "nobleman's son."

Ermin: *see* Herman.

Ernest: (Teutonic) "sincere; intent." Ernest Hemingway, writer. Also: **Earnest, Ernesto (Sp), Ernie.**

Errol: *see* Earl.

Erskine: a Scottish place name. Erskine Caldwell, writer.

Ervin, Erwin: *see* Irvin.

Esau: (Hebrew) "he that finishes." Biblical: son of Isaac, brother of Jacob.

Esmond: (Anglo-Saxon) "gracious protector."

Esteban: a Spanish form of Stephen.

Estes: (Latin) "from a famous ruling house."

Ethan: (Hebrew) "steadfast." Ethan Hawke, actor.
Also: **Etan.**

Ethelbert: *see* Albert.

Etheridge: (Teutonic) "gracious defender." Etheridge Knight, poet.

Etienne: French form of Stephen.

Eugene: (Greek) "noble; well-born." Eugene O'Neill, playwright.
Also: **Gene.**

Eustace: (Greek) "fruitful." St. Eustace, patron saint of hunters.
Also: **Eustacio (Sp).**

Evan: *see* John. Evans Carlson, U.S. Marine Corps general.

Evander: (Celtic) "young warrior." Evander Holyfield, boxer. Mythology: the son of Hermes.

Evelyn: (Old English) "a dear youth." Evelyn Waugh, novelist.

Everard: (Teutonic) "mighty as a boar."
Also: **Eberhart, Ev, Everett.**

Everett: *see* Everard. Everett Dirksen, U.S. senator.

Ewald: (Latin) "the bearer of good news."
Also: **Evald.**

Ewert: (Old English) "ewe herder."

Ewing: (Old English) "law friend."

Eynon: (Welsh) "anvil."

Ezekiel: (Hebrew) "God's strength." Biblical: the Book of Ezekiel. Ezekiel Cheever, 17th-century American schoolteacher.
Also: **Zeke.**

Ezra: (Hebrew) "the helper." Biblical: the Book of Ezra. Ezra Pound, poet.

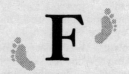

Fabian: (Latin) a Roman clan name.
Also: **Fabe, Fabiano, Fabien, Fabio.**

Fabio: *see* Fabian.

Fabrice, Fabron: (South French) "little blacksmith."
Also: **Fabrizio (It).**

Fagan: (Irish Gaelic) "little fiery one."

Fairfax: (Anglo-Saxon) "fair; yellow-haired." Fairfax Cone, advertising executive.

Fairley: (Anglo-Saxon) "from the fair meadow."
Also: **Fairlie, Farley.**

Falconer: *see* Falkner.

Falkner: (Anglo-Saxon) "falcon hunter; trainer."
Also: **Falconer, Faulkner, Fowler.**

Fallon: (Irish Gaelic) "of a ruling family."

Fane: (Old English) "glad; joyful."

Farand: (Teutonic) "attractive; pleasant."
Also: **Farant, Farrand, Ran.**

Fariid: (Muslim) "unique."

Farley: see Fairley. Farley Mowat, Canadian author of *Never Cry Wolf.*
Also: **Fairleigh.**

Farmer: (Teutonic) "one who tills the field."

Farnell: (Old English) "from the fern slope."
Also: **Fernald.**

Farnham: (Old English) "from the fern field."

Farnley: (Old English) "from the fern meadow."

Farold: (Old English) "mighty traveler."

Farr: (Old English) "traveler."

Farrand: see Farand.

Farrell: (Celtic) "the valorous one."
Also: **Farrel.**

Faulkner: see Falkner.

Faust: (Latin) "lucky, auspicious."
Also: **Faustino (Sp).**

Favian: (Latin) "a man of understanding."

Faxon: (Teutonic) "renowned for his hair."

Fay: (Irish Gaelic) "raven."

Fedor, Fedorico: see Theodore.

Felipe: a Spanish form of Philip.

Felix: (Latin) "fortunate." Felix Block, physicist.
Also: **Feliciano (Sp).**

Felton: (Old English) "from the field estate."

Fenton: (Anglo-Saxon) "dweller of the marshland."

Feodor: see Theodore.

Ferdinand: (Teutonic) "bold venture." Ferdinand II, king of Aragon.
Also: **Ferd, Ferde, Ferdie, Fernand, Fernando, Hernando.**

Fergus: (Celtic) "best choice; strong man." A legendary hero of Celtic lore.
Also: **Fergie, Ferguson.**

Fernald: see Farnell.

Fernando: see Ferdinand.

Ferris: (Celtic) "rock." Ferris Bueller, teenage protagonist of the film *Ferris Bueller's Day Off.*

Fidel: (Latin) "faithful."

Fielding: (Old English) "dweller at the field."

Filbert: (Old English) "very brilliant one." *See also* Philbert.

Filmer: (Old English) "very famous one."
Also: **Filmore.**

Filmore: see Filmer.

Findlay: see Finley.

Finley: (Irish Gaelic) "little fair-haired valorous one."
Also: **Findlay, Finlay.**

Finn: (Irish Gaelic) "Fair-haired and -complexioned." Finn Ronne, explorer.
Also: **Fynn.**

Firman: (Anglo-Saxon) "traveler to distant places."

Fisher: (English) "fisherman." Fisher Stevens, actor.
Also: **Fischer.**

Fisk: (Scandinavian) "the fisherman."
Also: **Fiske.**

Fitch: (Middle English) "European ermine or marten."

Fitzgerald: (Teutonic) "a son of Gerald."
Also: **Fitz.**

Fitzhugh: (Old English) "son of the intelligent one."

Fitzpatrick: (Teutonic) "a son of Patrick."

Flann: (Irish) "blood red."
Also: **Flanagan, Flannery, Flannigan.**

Flavian: (Latin) "fair; blond."
Also: **Flaviano (Sp), Flavius.**

Flavius: see Flavian.

Fleming: (Anglo-Saxon) "the Dutchman." Flemming Flindt, ballet choreographer.
Also: **Flem.**

Fletcher: (French) "arrow maker." Fletcher Christian, first mate in *Mutiny on the Bounty.*
Also: **Fletch.**

Flint: (English) "rock; flint."

Flip: see Philip.

Florian: (Latin) "flowering; blooming."
Also: **Florence, Florent, Flores, Florian, Floris, Flory.**

Floyd: see Lloyd.

Forbes: a Scottish place name.

Ford: see Bradford. Ford Maddox Ford, author.

Forrest: (Teutonic) "from the woods."
Also: **Forest, Forrester, Foster.**

Forrester: (Middle English) "forest guardian."
Also: **Forster.**

Fortune: (Old French) "lucky one."
Also: **Fortunato (It, Sp).**

Foster: (Teutonic) "forester; keeper of the preserve." Foster Brooks, comedian.
See also Forrest.

Fowler: see Falkner.

Fox: (English) "the fox."

Francesco: see Francis. Francesco Clemente, artist.

Francis: (Latin) from France. St. Francis of Assisi; Francis Ford Coppola, film director. Fran Tarkenton, quarterback.
Also: **Francesco (It), Franchot, Francisco (Sp), François (Fr), Frank, Frankie, Franz.**

Francisco: see Francis.

Frank: see Francis, Franklin.

Franklin: (Teutonic) "a free man." Franklin Chang-Diaz, first Hispanic-American in space.
Also: **Frank, Franklyn.**

Franz: see Francis.

Fraser: see Frazer.

Frayne: (Middle English) "stranger."

Frazer: (Old English) "curly-haired." (Old French) "strawberry."
Also: **Fraser, Frazier.**

Fred: see Frederick.

Frederick: (Teutonic) "peace-ful chieftain."
Also: **Federico, Fred, Freddie, Freddy, Frederic, Fredric, Fritz.**

Freeman: (Anglo-Saxon) "one born free."
Also: **Freemon.**

Fremont: (Old German) "free or noble protector."

Frewin: (Old English) "free, noble friend."

Frey: (Old English) "lord."

Frick: (Old English) "bold man."

Fridolf: (Old English) "peace-ful wolf."

Fritz: Fritz Lang, film director (1890–1976).
Also: **Friz.** *See also* Frederick.

Fuller: (Middle English) "cloth-thickener."

Fulton: (Anglo-Saxon) "from a field; farm town." Fulton Al-lem, golfer.

Fulvio: (Latin) "red-haired." Fulvio Testa, artist.

Furnell: the surname used as a first name. Furnell Chat-man, newscaster.

Fyfe: (Pictish-Scottish) from Fifeshire, Scotland.

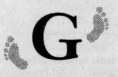

Gable: (Old French) "little Gabriel."
Also: **Gabel.**

Gabriel: (Hebrew) "God is mighty." Biblical: the arch-angel Gabriel. Gabriel García Márquez, Colombian author.
Also: **Gabby, Gabe.**

Gadman: (Hebrew) "the fortu-nate."
Also: **Gad, Gadmon.**

Gage: (Old French) "pledge."

Gaines: the English surname used as a first name.

Gair: (Irish Gaelic) "short one."

Gaius: (Latin) "to rejoice."
Also: **Cai, Caio, Caius.**

Gale: (Celtic) "lively." Gale Sayers, football player.
Also: **Gail, Gayle.**

Galen: (Greek) "healer." Ga-len Rowell, adventurer.
Also: **Gaelan.**

Gallagher: (Irish Gaelic) "ea-ger helper."
Also: **Gallaher.**

Galliard: (Old French) "jovial, merry."

Galloway: (Old Gaelic) "man from the land of Gaels."
Also: **Galway.**

Galton: (Old English) "owner of a rented estate."
Also: **Galt.**

Galvin: (Celtic) "the spar-row."
Also: **Vin, Vinny.**

Galway: a county and city in western Ireland. Galway Kinnell, poet.

Gamaliel: (Hebrew) "the Lord is my recompense." Biblical: the mentor of Paul. Gama-

liel Bradford, American biographer.

Gannon: (Irish Gaelic) "little fair-complexioned one."

Gar: diminutive of any name beginning with Gar-; also used as an independent name.

Garcia: (Spanish) "fox."

Gardiner: (Teutonic) "gardener."
Also: **Gardener, Gardner, Garth.**

Gareth: see Garett. One of King Arthur's knights.

Garett: (Welsh) "gentle."
Also: **Garet, Gareth, Garey, Garratt, Garret, Garreth, Garrett, Garry, Gary.**

Garey: see Garett.

Garfield: (Old English) "triangular field."
Also: **Garry, Gary.**

Garibald: (Old English) "a welcome addition."
Also: **Gary.**

Garland: (Old English) "from the spear land."
Also: **Garlen.**

Garman: (Old English) "spearman."
Also: **Garmon.**

Garmond: (Old English) "spear protector."

Garner: (Teutonic) "the defender; noble guardian."

Garnet: (Latin) "grain; red jewel." Sir Garnet Wolseley, founder of the modern British army.
Also: **Garnett.**

Garnock: (Old Welsh) "dweller by the alder tree."

Garret: see Garett.

Garrick: (Teutonic) "mighty warrior." Garrick Olson, pianist.
Also: **Gerik, Rick.**

Garrison: (Teutonic) "fortified." Garrison Keillor, radio personality, author.
Also: **Garson.**

Garroway: (Old English) "spear warrior."

Garson: (French) "garrison." Garson Kanin, screenwriter.

Garth: (Anglo-Saxon) a form of Gardener. Garth Brooks, country singer.

Garton: (Old English) "dweller at the triangular farmstead."

Garvey: (Irish Gaelic) "rough peace."

Garvin: (Teutonic) "battle friend."
Also: **Gar, Gary.**

Garwood: (Old English) "from the fir forest."

Gary: see Garett, Garvin.

Gaspar, Gaspard: see Jasper.

Gaston: (Teutonic) from Gascony. Gaston Lachaise, sculptor.
Also: **Gascon.**

Gavin: see Gawain. Gavin Stevens, Southern lawyer protagonist in series of Faulkner short stories.

Gawain: (Teutonic) "hawk; falcon." Literary: the Arthurian hero Sir Gawain.
Also: **Gavin.**

Gaylord: (Anglo-Saxon) "the joyous nobleman." Gaylord Perry, baseball pitcher.

Gaynor: (Irish Gaelic) "son of the fair-head."

Geary: (Middle English) "changeable one."

Geber: (Hebrew) "strong."

Gebhard: (Teutonic) "a generous person."
Also: **Gebhardt, Gebhart.**

Genaro: (Latin) "born in January."

Gene: see Eugene.

Geng: (Chinese) "the seventh of the Ten Heavenly Stems." Traditionally combined with another name.

Geoffrey: (Teutonic) "God's peace; peace of the land." Geoffrey Beene, fashion designer.
Also: **Geof, Geoff, Godfrey, Jeff, Jeffers, Jeffery, Jeffrey.**

George: (Greek) "farmer; tiller of the soil." St. George, the patron saint of England.
Also: **Geordie, Georgy, Giorgio (It), Jerzy (Pol), Jorge (Sp).**

Gerald: (Teutonic) "mighty spearman." Gerald Carr, astronaut.
Also: **Garold, Geraldo (Sp), Gerard (Fr), Gereld, Gerrald, Gerry, Gery, Jereld, Jerold, Jerrold, Jerry.**

Gerard: see Gerald.

Gerhard: (Teutonic) "hardy fighter."
Also: **Gerhart.**

Germaine: (Latin) "a German."
Also: **Jermaine.**

Geronimo: see Jerome. Geronimo, Apache chief.

Gerry: see Garett, Gerald, Jermyn.

Gervase: (Teutonic) "spear vassal; honorable."
Also: **Gervaise, Gervasio (Sp), Jarv, Jarvey, Jarvis, Jervis.**

Gian: see John.

Gibson: (Old English) "son of Gilbert."
Also: **Gibbs.**

Gideon: (Hebrew) "brave warrior; indomitable spirit." Biblical: judge of Israel.

Gifford: (Teutonic) "gift." Gifford Pinchot, conservationist.

Gil: short form for names beginning Gil-.

Gilad: (Hebrew) "man from Giladi."
Also: **Gil.**

Gilbert: (Teutonic) "bright pledge."
Also: **Gil, Gilberto (Sp), Gilpin.**

Gilby: (Old Norse) "hostage's estate."

Gilchrist: (Irish Gaelic) "servant of Christ."

Gilder: "one who gilds."

Giles: (Latin) "shield bearer."
Also: **Gil, Gile, Gilles, Gilly, Gyles.**

Gillian: (Celtic) "servant of the saints."
Also: **Gillean.**

Gilmer: (Old English) "famous hostage."

Gilmore: (Irish Gaelic) "adherent of St. Mary."

Gilroy: (Latin) "the king's faithful servant."

Giorgio: Italian form of George.

Giovanni: Italian form of John.

Girvin: (Irish Gaelic) "little rough one."

Glade: (Old English) "shining."
Also: **Gladney, Gladstone.**

Gladwin: *see* Goodwin.

Glanville: (Old French) "from the oak-tree estate."

Glen: (Celtic) "from the valley."
Also: **Glenn, Glynn.**

Glendon: (Teutonic) "dweller in the dark glen."
Also: **Glennard.**

Glover: (Teutonic) "one who makes gloves."

Goddard: (Teutonic) "of a firm nature."
Also: **Godderd, Goddord.**

Godfrey: a variant of Geoffrey.

Godwin: (Old English) "God; friend."

Golan: (Hebrew) "passage; revolution." An Israeli place name.

Golding: (Old English) "golden."

Goldwin: (Old English) "golden friend."

Gomer: (Hebrew) "to finish, complete."

Gonzales, Gonzalez: the Spanish surname.

Goodman: (Teutonic) "good man."

Goodwin: (Teutonic) "good and faithful friend."
Also: **Gladwin, Godwin.**

Gordon: (Anglo-Saxon) "from the cornered hill." Gordie Howe, hockey great.
Also: **Gorden, Gordy.**

Gorman: (Irish-Gaelic) "little blue-eyed one."

Gouverneur: (French) "governor."

Gowell: (Norse) "gold." Also a type of daisy.

Gower: (Old Welsh) "pure one." Gower Champion, choreographer.

Gracian: (Latin) "graceful."
Also: **Graciano.**

Grady: (Irish Gaelic) "noble; illustrious."

Graham: (Teutonic) "from the gray home."
Also: **Graeme, Grahame, Ham.**

Granger: (Old English) "farmer."
Also: **Grange.**

Grant: (French) "grand." Grant Hill, basketball player; Grant Wood, artist.

Grantland: (Old English) "from the great grassy plain." Grantland Rice, sportswriter.

Granville: (French) "of the big town." Granville Hall, psychologist.
Also: **Grenville.**

Grayson: (Old English) "a judge's son."

Also: **Gray, Graydon, Grey, Greyson.**

Greeley: (Old English) "from the gray meadow."

Greg: see Gregory.

Gregory: (Greek) "vigilant." St. Gregory of Nyssa; Gregor Mendel, botanist.
Also: **Greg, Gregg, Gregorio (It, Sp).**

Gresham: (Anglo-Saxon) "from the grazing land."

Griffin: see Griffith. In Greek mythology the griffin was a creature with the body of a lion and the head and wings of an eagle. Griffin Dunne, actor, director.

Griffith: (Celtic) "red-haired."
Also: **Griff, Griffin, Rufus.**

Griswold: (Teutonic) "from the wild gray forest."

Grover: (Anglo-Saxon) "grove-dweller." Grover Cleveland, 22nd and 24th U.S. President.
Also: **Grove.**

Guido: see Guy.

Guillaume: French form of William.
Also: **Guillermo (Sp).**

Guion: (origin uncertain) Guion Bluford, the first black American in space.

Gunnar: see Gunther.

Gunther: (Teutonic) "bold warrior."
Also: **Gunar, Gunnar, Guntar, Gunter, Gunthar.**

Gus: see Angus, Argus, August, Gustave.

Gustave: (Scandinavian) "noble staff." Gustave Flaubert, author.
Also: **Gus, Gustaf, Gustavus.**

Gustin: see August.

Guthrie: (Celtic) "war hero."

Guy: (Teutonic) "lively."
Also: **Guido, Guyon, Wiatt, Wyatt.**

Gwyn: (Welsh) "fair." Gwyn Thomas, Welsh novelist.
Also: **Gwynn, Gwynne.**

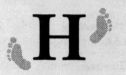

Hackett: (Old Franco-German) "little woodsman."

Hadar: (Hebrew) "ornament; splendor."

Haden: (Old English) "of the moors."
Also: **Hadden, Haddon.**

Hadley: (Old English) "from the heath meadow."
Also: **Hadleigh.**

Hadrian: see Adrian.

Hadwin: (Old English) "war-friend."

Hagen: (Irish Gaelic) "little; young one."

Hagley: (Old English) "from the hedged pasture."

Haig: (Old English) "dweller at the hedged enclosure."

Haima: (Sanskrit) "made of gold."

Haines: (Teutonic) "from a vined cottage."
Also: **Haynes.**

Haji: (Arabic) "pilgrim."

Hakim, Hakeem: (Arabic) "judge." Hakeem Olajuwon, basketball player.

Hakon: (Old Norse) "of the high race."

Hal: see Harold, Henry.

Halbert: (Old English) "brilliant hero."

Halden: (Teutonic) "half Dane." Haldan Hartline, biophysicist.
Also: **Haldane.**

Haldsey: (Anglo-Saxon) "from Hal's island."
Also: **Halsy.**

Hale: (Old English) "from the hall." Hale Irwin, golfer.

Haley: (English) "hay meadow."
Also: **Hayley.**

Halford: (Old English) "from the hill-slope ford."

Hall: (Old English) "from the master's house; stone."

Hallet: (Old English) "dweller at the little manor."

Halley: (Old English) "from the manor-house meadow."

Halliwell: (Old English) "dweller by a holy spring."

Hallward: (Old English) "hall warden."

Halstead: (Old English) "from the manor-house place."

Halton: (Old English) "from the hill-slope estate."

Hamal: (Arabic) "lamb."

Hamar: (Old Norse) "a symbol of ingenuity."

Hamilton: (French) "from the mountain hamlet." Hamilton Fish, American statesman.

Hamish: see James.

Hamlet: (Old Franco-German) "little home." Literary: Shakespeare's Prince of Denmark.

Hamlin, Hamlyn: see Henry. Hamlin Garland, Pulitzer prize–winning author.

Han: (Chinese) "Chinese; male; self-restraint." Traditionally combined with another name.

Hanford: (Old English) "from the high ford."

Hank: see Henry.

Hanley: (Anglo-Saxon) "of the high meadow."
Also: **Hanleigh, Henleigh, Henley, Henry.**

Hannibal: Hannibal, the Carthaginian general.

Hans: see John. Hans Christian Andersen, Danish writer of fairy tales.
Also: **Hansen.**

Hansel: (Scandinavian) "a gift from the Lord."

Hansen, Hanson: (Scandinavian) "son of Hans."

Harald: see Harold.

Haran: (Hebrew) "mountainous country."

Harbert: see Herbert.

Harbin: (Old Franco-German) "small, glorious warrior."

Harcourt: (French) "from an armed court."

Harden: (Old English) "from the hare valley."

Harding: (Old English) "brave one's son."
Also: **Hardy.**

Hardwin: (Old English) "brave friend."

Hardy: (Teutonic) "of hardy stock."
Also: **Hardie.**

Harford: (Old English) "from the hare ford."

Hargrove: (Old English) "from the hare grove."
Also: **Hargrave.**

Harlan: (Teutonic) "from the battle land." Harlan Ellison, writer.
Also: **Harland.**

Harley: (Anglo-Saxon) "from the hare's or stag's meadow." Harley Granville-Barker, Edwardian English actor, dramatist.
Also: **Arley, Arlie, Harden, Harleigh, Hart, Hartley.**

Harlow: (Old English) "fortified hill."

Harman, Harmon: see Herman. Harmon Killebrew, baseball player.

Harod: (Hebrew) "the loud terror."
Also: **Harrod.**

Harold: (Anglo-Saxon) "army commander." Harold Prince, theatrical producer, director.
Also: **Hal, Harald, Harry, Herald, Hereld, Herold, Herrick.**

Harper: (Old English) "harp player." Harper Lee, author of *To Kill a Mockingbird.*

Harris, Harrison: (Old English) "son of Henry/Harry." Harrison Ford, actor.

Harry: see Harold, Henry.

Hart: (Old English) "hart deer." Hart Crane, poet. *See also* Harley, Hartwell.

Hartford: (Old English) "stag ford." Hartford Gunn, founder of the Public Broadcasting Service.

Hartley: see Harley.

Hartman: (Old German) "strong man."

Hartwell: (Teutonic) "from the deer's spring."
Also: **Hart, Harwell, Harwill.**

Hartwood: (Old English) "hart deer forest."
Also: **Harwood.**

Harvey: (French) "bitter."
Also: **Harv, Harve, Herv, Herve, Hervey.**

Hasan: (Arabic) "handsome."
Also: **Hassan.**

Haskell: (Hebrew) "wisdom; understanding." Haskell Wexler, cinematographer.

Haslett: (Old English) "hazel-tree headland."

Hastings: (Old English) "son of the violent one."

Hatcher: (Old English) "a small wasteland." Hatcher Hughes, Pulitzer prize–winning dramatist.

Havelock: (Old Norse) "seaport."

Haven: (English) "place of refuge."

Hawk: Also: **Hawke.**

Hawley: (Old English) "from the hedged meadow."

Hawthorne: place name referring to the hawthorn tree; surname of Nathaniel Hawthorne, author.

Hayden: (Teutonic) "from the hedged hill."
Also: **Haydn, Haydon.**

Hayes: (Old English) "from the woods; the hunter." Hayes Jenkins, champion ice skater.

Hayley: see Haley.

Hayward: (Old English) "hedged-enclosure keeper."

Haywood: (Old English) "from the hedged forest."
Also: **Heywood.**

Heath: (Anglo-Saxon) "from the vast wasteland."
Also: **Heathbrook.**

Heathcliff: (Middle English) "from the heath cliff." Heathcliff, brooding hero of Emily Brontë's *Wuthering Heights.*
Also: **Cliff, Heath.**

Hector: (Greek) "steady; unswerving." Mythology: Hector was a hero of the Trojan War. Hector Babenco, film director.

Hedley: "a clearing where heather grows." Hedley Donovan, publishing executive.

Heinrick, Hendrick, Hendrik: see Henry.

Heliodoro: (Greek/Spanish) "the sun." Helios, the Greek sun god.
Also: **Elio, Helio.**

Heller: German form of Helio.

Helmar: (Teutonic) "famous warrior."

Henderson: (English) "son of Henry."

Henley: see Hanley.

Henry: (Teutonic) "home ruler."
Also: **Enrico (It), Enrique (Sp), Hal, Hamlin, Hank, Harry, Heinrick, Hendrick, Hendrik, Henri (Fr).** See also Hanley, Harris.

Herald: see Harold.

Herbert: (Teutonic) "bright warrior."
Also: **Bert, Harbert, Herb, Hilbert.**

Herman, Hermann: (Teutonic) "noble warrior." Herman Melville, author.
Also: **Armand (Fr), Armando (Sp), Armin, Armond, Armyn, Ermin, Harman, Harmon, Herm, Hermon.**

Hermes: in Greek mythology, Hermes was the messenger of the gods.

Hernando: see Ferdinand.

Herrick: (Old German) "army ruler." See also Harold.

Herrod: (Hebrew) "heroic conqueror."
Also: **Herod.**

Herschel: (Hebrew) "deer."

Herschel Walker, football player.
Also: **Hershel.**

Hervey: see Harvey.

Herwin: (Teutonic) "a friend; lover of battle."

Hewe: see Hugh.

Hewett: (Old Franco-German) "little Hugh."
Also: **Hewitt.**

Heywood: see Haywood.

Hezekiah: (Hebrew) "God is strength." Biblical: king of Judah.
Also: **Hesketh.**

Hi: diminutive of Hiram, Hilary, and Hyman.

Hiatt: see Hyatt.

Hickory: an American name from nature.

Hilary: (Latin) "cheerful; merry." Saint Hilary of Poitiers.
Also: **Hilaire, Hillary.**

Hildebrand: (Old German) "war sword."

Hillel: (Hebrew) "greatly praised."

Hilliard: (Teutonic) "war guardian; protector."
Also: **Hillard.**

Hilman: (English) "dweller on a hill."

Hilton: (Old English) "from the house on the hill."

Hinman: (Teutonic) "one who serves."

Hinton: (English) "homestead on high land." Hinton Battle, actor.

Hiram: (Hebrew) "most no-ble; exalted." Biblical: the king of Tyre. Hiram Revels, the first black senator.
Also: **Hy.**

Hiroshi: (hee-ROW-shee) (Japanese) "peaceful; spacious; plentiful." Hiro, fashion photographer.

Hiwa: (Hawaiian) the color clear black.

Hoagland: (Swiss) "high grove." Hoagy Carmichael, songwriter (1899–1981).

Hobart: see Hubert. Hobie Alter, "Hobie Cat" sailboat designer.

Hodge, Hodgekin: diminutives of Roger.

Hogan: (Irish Gaelic) "youth."

Holbrook: (Anglo-Saxon) "from the valley brook."

Holcomb: (Old English) "deep valley."

Holden: (Teutonic) "kind." Holden Caulfield, young protagonist of J. D. Salinger's novel The Catcher in the Rye.

Holger: (Scandinavian) "noble spear."

Holland: (Dutch) "woodland." Place name used as a first name.

Hollis: (Anglo-Saxon) "dweller by the holly trees."

Holmes: (Middle English) "from the river islands."
Also: **Holm.**

Holt: (Old English) "from the forest." Holt Marvel, jazz artist.

Homer: (Greek) "pledge."

Also, the name of the poet used as a first name.

Honor: *see* Honorius. Honor Arundel, author.

Honorius: (Latin) "man of honor." Honorius, Roman emperor.
Also: **Honor.**

Horace: (Latin) "timekeeper." Horace Greeley, American journalist.
Also: **Horatio, Horatius, Race.**

Horatio: *see* Horace. Horatio Alger, writer.

Horton: (Old English) "from the gray estate." Horton Foote, dramatist.
Also: **Horten.**

Hosea: (Hebrew) "salvation." Biblical: the Book of Hosea.

Houghton: (Old English) "from the estate on the bluff."

Houston: (Anglo-Saxon) "from a mountain town"; the Texas city. Houston Baker, Jr., educator.
Also: **Huston.**

Howard: (Teutonic) "chief guardian."

Howe: (Old German) "eminent one."

Howell: (Old Welsh) "eminent; conspicuous."
Also: **Hywel.**

Howland: (Old English) "of the hills."

Hoyt: *see* Hubert. Hoyt Axton, country singer.

Hu: (Chinese) "tiger; amber." Traditionally combined with another name. Hu Shi, Chinese ambassador to the U.S.

Hubert: (Teutonic) "shining of mind."
Also: **Hobart, Hoyt, Hubbard, Hubie.**

Hudson: (English) "son of Hudde."

Hugh: (Teutonic) "mind; intelligence."
Also: **Hewe, Huey, Hughes, Hughie, Hugo (Pol), Ugo (It).**

Hugo: *see* Hugh.

Humbert: (Teutonic) "bright home."
Also: **Bert, Bertie, Umberto (It).**

Hume: (Teutonic) "lover of his home." Hume Cronyn, actor.

Humphrey: (Teutonic) "a protector of the peace." Humphrey Bogart, actor.
Also: **Humfrey.**

Hunter: (Old English) "the hunter." Hunter S. Thompson, writer.
Also: **Hunt, Huntley.**

Huntington: (Old English) "hunting estate." Huntington Hartford, businessman.
Also: **Huntingdon.**

Huntley: (Old English) "from the hunter's meadow." *See also* Hunter.

Hurlbert: (Old English) "brilliant army leader."

Hurley: (Irish Gaelic) "sea tide."

Hurst: (Middle English) "dweller at the forest."
Also: **Hearst.**

Huston: *see* Houston. Huston Smith, religious scholar.

Hutton: (Old English) "from the estate on the projecting ridge."

Huxford: (Old English) "Hugh's ford."

Huxley: (Old English) "Hugh's meadow."

Hy: diminutive of Hiram, Hilary, and Hyman.

Hyatt: (Old English) "from the high gate."
Also: **Hiatt.**

Hyde: (Old English) "from the acreage that supported one family."

Hyman: (Hebrew) "life." Masculine of Eve.
Also: **Chaim, Hy.**

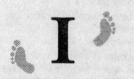

Ian: Scottish form of John. Ian Fleming, James Bond author.
Also: **Iain.**

Ibrahim: Muslim form of Abraham.

Ichabod: (Hebrew) "the glory has departed."

Ignatius: (Latin) "the fiery and ardent." St. Ignatius Loyola, founder of the Jesuits.
Also: **Iggy, Ignace, Ignacio (Sp), Ignatz.**

Igor: (Russian) "Ing's warrior." Igor Stravinsky, composer.
Also: **Inge, Ingmar.**

Ike: a form of Isaac.

Ilias: (Greek-Latin) the ancient name of Troy, giving title to Homer's epic *Iliad.*

Illinois: the state of Illinois, named by the Indians, who called themselves Iliniwek, "true admirable men." Illinois Jacquet, jazz artist.

Immanuel: *see* Emmanuel.

Indiana: Indiana State, so named because it was purchased by the U.S. from the Indians in 1795. Indiana Jones, adventuring archaeologist of the movie *Raiders of the Lost Ark.*

Indra: (Hindustani) "god of the thunderstorm." Indra is the warrior god of Indian mythology.

Ingalls: (English) "Ing's tribute."

Inglebert: (Old German) "brilliant angel."

Ingmar: a form of Ingvar. Ingmar Bergman, film director.

Ingram: (Teutonic) "the raven."
Also: **Ingraham.**

Ingvar: (Norse) "Ing's warrior."

Inir: (Welsh) "honor."

Innes: (Celtic) "from the island."
Also: **Innis.**

Ion: a variant of Ian.

Ira: (Hebrew) "watcher." Ira Gershwin, lyricist.

Irvin: (Anglo-Saxon) "sea friend."
Also: **Earvin, Ervin, Ervine, Erwin, Irv, Irving, Irwin, Marv, Marvin, Merv, Mervin, Merwin.**

Irving: *see* Irvin. Irving Berlin, songwriter.

Irwin: *see* Irvin.

Isaac: (Hebrew) "laughing." Biblical: the son of Abraham. Isaac Asimov, science fiction writer.
Also: **Ike, Itzaak, Izaac, Izzy.**

Isaiah: (Hebrew) "salvation of the Lord." Biblical: the prophet Isaiah. Isaiah Thomas, patriot of the American Revolution.

Isamu: (EE-saw-moo) (Japanese) "brave, courageous." Isamu Noguchi, sculptor.

Isao: (EE-saw-oh) (Japanese) "merit, achievement." Isao Aoki, golfer.

Isham: (Old English) "from the iron one's estate."

Ishmael: (Hebrew) "God will hear." Ishmael Reed, poet.

Isidore: (Greek) "a gift." Saint Isidore of Seville; Isidor Stone, journalist.
Also: **Dore, Dorian, Dory, Isador, Isadore, Isidor, Isidro (Sp), Issy, Iz, Izzy.**

Isman: (Hebrew) "a loyal husband."

Israel: (Hebrew) "the Lord's warrior; soldier." Biblical: the name given to Jacob by God.
Also: **Issy, Iz, Izzy.**

Italo: (Latin) "Italian." Italo Calvino, author.

Itzaak: *see* Isaac.

Ivan: a Russian form of John.
Also: **Varek.**

Ivar: a form of Ingvar.
Also: **Iver, Ives, Ivo, Ivon, Ivor, Yves.**

Iven: (Old French) "little yew-bow."

Ives: *see* Ivar, Yves.

Ivor: variant of Ingvar.

Izaac, Izzy: *see* Isaac.

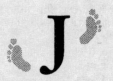

J

Jaafar: (Arabic) "small river."
Also: **Jafar.**

Jabez: (Hebrew) "cause of sorrow."
Also: **Jabe.**

Jacinto: (Greek) "hyacinth flower." Jacinto Benavente, Nobel prize–winning dramatist.

Jack: *see* James, John.

Jackson: (Old English) "son of Jack." Jackson Browne, singer, songwriter; Jackson Pollock, artist.

Jacob: *see* James. Biblical: son of Isaac and Rebecca, husband of Leah and Rachel. The twelve tribes of Israel evolved from Jacob's twelve sons.
Also: **Jacobo (Sp), Jacques (Fr), Jake.**

Jacques: French form of James. Jacques Cousteau, scientist.

Jael: (Hebrew) "he that ascends."

Jagger: (North English) "carter; teamster."

Jamal, Jamaal: (Arabic) "elegance; beauty."
Also: **Jamel.**

James: (Hebrew) "the supplanter." Biblical: the name of two apostles.
Also: **Diego, Hamish, Jack, Jacob, Jacques, Jaime (Sp), Jake, Jakie, Jameson, Jamesy, Jamie, Jayme, Jem, Jemmie, Jemmy, Jim, Jimmie, Jimmy, Jock, Jocko, Seamus, Shamus.**

Jamie: a form of James. Jamie Wyeth, American painter.

Jan: (yahn) Dutch form of John. Jann Wenner, publisher.

Janssen: (Scandinavian) "John's son."

Jantu: (Sanskrit) "male child."

Janus: (Latin) "a gate, passageway." Janus was the Roman god of beginnings and endings. The first month of the year is named for him.

Jared: (Hebrew) "the descending; descendant."
Also: **Jareth, Jarod, Jered, Jarrad.**

Jarlath: (Latin) "man of control."

Jarman: (Old German) "the German."

Jarvis: see Gervase.

Jason: (Greek) "healer." Mythology: leader of the Argonauts.
Also: **Jayson.**

Jasper: (Persian) "treasure bringer." Also a semiprecious stone. The English name of one of the three Magi. Jasper Johns, American painter.
Also: **Casper, Cass, Gaspar, Gaspard (Fr), Kaspar.**

Javier: see Xavier.

Jay, Jaye: (Anglo-Saxon) "the jaybird." Also used as a diminutive for names beginning with J. Stephen Jay Gould, paleontologist.

Jean: French form of John. Jean Piaget, psychologist.

Jeconiah: (Hebrew) "gift of the Lord."

Jed: see Jedediah.

Jedediah: (Hebrew) "beloved by the Lord." Jedediah Smith, 19th-century explorer.
Also: **Jed, Jeddy, Jedidiah.**

Jeevan: (Hindi) "life."

Jefferson: (Old English) "son of Jeffrey." Jefferson Davis, president of the Confederate states.

Jeffrey: see Geoffrey.

Jegar: (Hebrew) "witness our love."
Also: **Jeggar, Jegger.**

Jerald, Jerold, Jerrold: see Gerald.

Jeremiah: (Hebrew) "exalted by the Lord." Biblical: the

Book of Jeremiah. *See also* Jeremy.

Jeremy: a form of Jeremiah. Jeremy Irons, actor.
Also: **Jeremias, Jerry.**

Jericho: (English) "his moon or month." The biblical place name.

Jermaine: *see* Jermyn.

Jermyn: (Latin) "a German."
Also: **Germaine, Gerry, Jermaine, Jerry.**

Jerome: (Greek) "holy." Saint Jerome; Jerome Kern, composer.
Also: **Geronimo, Jerry.**

Jerry: familiar form of Gerald and names beginning Ger- and Jer-.

Jervis: *see* Gervase.

Jesse: (Hebrew) "God's gift; grace." Biblical: the father of King David. Jesse Owens, Olympic track star.
Also: **Jess.**

Jesus: *see* Joshua.

Jethro: (Hebrew) "outstanding; excellent." Biblical: the father-in-law of Moses.
Also: **Jeth.**

Jett: from Jet, a black gemstone.

Jevon: *see* John.

Ji: (Chinese) "foundation; discipline; achievement; continuity." Traditionally combined with a second name.

Jian: (Chinese) "solid; to build." Traditionally combined with a second name.

Jim: *see* James.

Joab: (Hebrew) "praise the Lord." Biblical: commander under King David.

Joachim, Joachin: (Hebrew) "the Lord will judge." Joachin Phoenix, actor; Joachin Miller, poet.

Job: (Hebrew) "the persecuted; the afflicted." Biblical: the Book of Job.
Also: **Joby.**

Jock: *see* James, John.

Jody: a contemporary name.

Joe, Joey: *see* Joseph.

Joel: (Hebrew) "Jehovah is God." Biblical: a common Old Testament name, borne by 12 different characters.

Johan, Johann: *see* John.

John: (Hebrew) "God's gracious gift." Biblical: John the Baptist.
Also: **Evan, Gian, Giovanni (It), Hans, Ian, Ivan (Russ), Jack, Jan, Jean (Fr), Jevon, Jock, Johan, Johann, Johnnie, Johnny, Johnson, Jonnie, Jonny, Jon, Juan (Sp), Sean, Shane, Shawn, Zane.**

Jonah: *see* Jonas. Biblical: the father of Simon Peter.

Jonas: (Hebrew) "dove." Biblical: the Book of Jonah. Jonas Salk, scientist who developed the polio vaccine.
Also: **Jonah, Jone.**

Jonathan: (Hebrew) "gift of God." Biblical: the son of King Saul.
Also: **Jon.**

Jordan: (Hebrew) "flowing down." Biblical: the River

Jordan, where Jesus was baptized.
Also: **Jordie, Jourdan.**

Jorge: Spanish form of George.

Jorim: "he that exalts the Lord."
Also: **Joram.**

Joseph: (Hebrew) "He shall add." In the Old Testament Joseph is the beloved son of the patriarch Jacob, by whom he is given the coat of many colors. In the New Testament Joseph is the husband of Mary.
Also: **Giuseppe (It), Joe, Joey, Josef (German), Jose (Sp), Josef (Pol), Yusef (Arabic).**

Joshua: (Hebrew) "whom God has saved." Biblical: the commander who led the Israelites in the conquest of the Promised Land.
Also: **Jesus (Sp), Josh.**

Josiah: (Hebrew) "he is healed by the Lord." Josiah Bartlett, member of Continental Congress. Biblical: a king of Judah.
Also: **Jos, Josh.**

Jotham: (Hebrew) "God is perfect." Biblical: a king of Judah.
Also: **Joe.**

Joyner: (French) "to join together; carpenter."

Juan: Spanish form of John. Juan Gris, artist.

Judah: (Hebrew) "praise." Biblical: the fourth of Jacob's 12 sons. Judas, Judd, Juddah, Jude.

Judd: *see* Judah.

Jude: variant of Judah.

Judge: (English) "a judge." Judge Reinhold, actor.

Judson: (Teutonic) "the son of Judd."

Jules: *see* Julius.

Julian: *see* Julius. Julian Bond, civil rights leader.

Julio: Spanish form of Julius.

Julius: (Latin) "divinely youthful." Jule Stein, composer; Julius Erving, basketball player.
Also: **Joliet, Jules, Juley, Julian, Julie, Julio (Sp).**

Juma: (Arabic/Swahili) "born on Friday." Juma Ikangaa, long-distance runner.

Jun: (joon) (Japanese) "pure, sincere." Junichiro Tanizaki, writer.

Junius: (Latin) "born in June."
Also: **June, Junie.**

Jurgen: *see* George.

Justin: (Latin) "the just." Justinian the Great, Byzantine emperor.
Also: **Just, Juston, Justus, Justyn.**

Justis: (Old French) "justice."
Also: **Justice.**

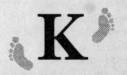

K

Kai: (Hawaiian) "the sea." Kai Krause, software designer.

Kalil: (Arabic) "good friend." Khalil Gibran, philosopher.

Kalton: (Greek) "beautiful town."

Kamal: (Arabic) "perfection." Also: **Kamali, Kamil.**

Kane: (Celtic) "bright; radiant."
Also: **Kayne.**

Kareem, Karim: (Arabic) "noble." Kareem Abdul-Jabbar, basketball player.

Karl: (German) "manly." Karel Reisz, film director.
Also: **Karle, Karlton, Karol, Karolek.** *See also* Carl.

Karsten: (Slavic) "Christian."

Kaspar: *see* Jasper.

Kay: (Latin) "rejoiced in." Also used as a diminutive for names beginning with K.

Keane: (Middle English) "bold, sharp one."
Also: **Kean.**

Keanu: (KEY-ah-noo) (Hawaiian) "cool breeze over the mountains." Keanu Reeves, actor.

Kearny: (Irish) "warlike; victorious."

Kedar: (Arabic) "powerful."

Keefe: (Irish Gaelic) "handsome; noble; gentle; lovable."

Keegan: (Irish Gaelic) "little fiery one."

Keelan: (Irish Gaelic) "little slender one."

Keeley: (Irish Gaelic) "handsome."

Keenan: (Irish Gaelic) "little ancient one." Keenan Wynn, actor.

Keiji: (KAY-gee) (Japanese) "joyous, happy."
Also: **Kei.**

Keiki: (KAY-kee) (Hawaiian) "child."

Keir: (Scottish) "a fort." Keir Dullea, actor.

Keith: a Scottish place name.

Kell: (Old Norse) "from the spring."

Keller: (Irish Gaelic) "little companion."

Kelly: (Irish Gaelic) "warrior."
Also: **Keeley, Kelly.**

Kelsey: (Teutonic) "from the water."
Also: **Kelcey.** Kelsey Grammer, television actor.

Kelvin: (Irish Gaelic) "from the narrow river."
Also: **Kel.**

Kemp: (Middle English) "champion."
Also: **Kemper.**

Ken: *see* Kenneth.

Kendall: (Celtic) "valley of the river Kent."
Also: **Kendell.**

Kendrick: (Anglo-Saxon) "royal ruler."
Also: **Ken, Kendricks, Kenrick.**

Kenelm: (Anglo-Saxon) "brave helmet."
Also: **Ken.**

Kenichi, Ken, Kenji: (Japanese) "wise; good health." Kenji Mizoguchi, film director (1898–1956).

Kenley: (Old English) "of the king's meadow."
Also: **Kenleigh.**

Kennard: (Old English) "bold, strong."

Kennedy: (Celtic) "chief of the clan."

Kenneth: (Celtic) "handsome."
Also: **Ken, Kennet, Kenny, Kent.**

Kenrick: (Old English) "bold ruler."

Kent: an English place name and surname.

Kenton: (Old English) "from the royal estate."

Kenward: (Old English) "bold guardian."

Kenway: (Anglo-Saxon) "the brave soldier."
Also: **Ken, Kenny.**

Kenwood: (Celtic) "wooded dell."

Kenya: (African) "artist." Also a contemporary place name. Kenya Wilkins, basketball player.

Kenyon: (Celtic) "fair-haired."
Also: **Ken, Kenny.**

Kerby: see Kirby.

Kermit: (Celtic) "free." The thoughtful frog Kermit of Muppets fame.
Also: **Dermot, Kerry.**

Kern: (Irish Gaelic) "little dark one."

Kerr: a Scottish surname.
Also: **Kerrie, Kerrin, Kerry, Kieran.** See also Kirby.

Kerrigan: an Irish surname. Kerrigan Mahan, theatre director.

Kerry: an Irish place name.

Kerry Kittles, basketball player.

Kerwin: (Irish Gaelic) "little jet-black one."
Also: **Kirwin.**

Kester: see Christopher.

Kevin: (Celtic) "kind; gentle."
Also: **Kev, Kevan.**

Key: (Irish Gaelic) "son of the fiery one."

Khalil: see Kalil.

Kieran: (Irish Gaelic) "little dark one." The name of 15 Irish saints.
Also: **Keira, Kerr, Kiera, Kieren, Kieron.**

Killian: (Irish Gaelic) "warlike."

Kim: (Vietnamese) "gold, metal." See also Kimball.

Kimball: (Anglo-Saxon) "royally brave." The name Kim comes from the Rudyard Kipling novel.
Also: **Kemble, Kim, Kimble.**

King: (Anglo-Saxon) "king." Kingman Brewster, president of Yale University.

Kingsley: (Anglo-Saxon) "from the king's meadow." Kingsley Amis, British author.
Also: **Kinsley.**

Kingston: (Old English) "dweller at the king's estate."

Kingswell: (Old English) "dweller at the king's spring."

Kinnard: (Irish Gaelic) "from the high hill."

Kinnell: (Irish Gaelic) "from the head of the cliff."

Kinsey: (Old English) "victorious one."

Kipp: (North English) "dweller at the pointed hill." Kip Keino, Olympic track athlete.

Kirby: (Teutonic) "from the church village."
Also: **Kerby, Kerr.**

Kirk: (Scandinavian) "of the church; living close to the church." Kirk Douglas, actor.
Also: **Kerk.**

Kirkland: (Scandinavian) "dweller on the church land."

Kirkley: (Old North English) "from the church meadow."

Kirkwood: (Old North English) "from the church forest."

Kirwin: see Kerwin.

Kit: see Christian, Christopher.

Klaus: see Nicholas.

Knight: (Middle English) "soldier."

Knox: (Old English) "from the hills."

Knute: (Danish) "from Canute, king of England and Denmark." Knute Rockne, football player, coach.

Konrad: see Conrad.

Kornel: variant of Cornell.

Kramer: (German) "tradesman."

Krishna: (Hindi) "delightful."

Kurt: see Curtis.

Kweisi: (Ghanan) "born on Sunday." Kweisi Mfume, congressman.

Kyle: (Gaelic) "a narrow piece of land." Kyle Rasmussen, skier.
Also: **Kile.**

Kynan: see Conal.

Kyne: (Old English) "royal one."

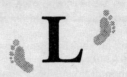

Laban: (Hebrew) "white." Biblical: father of Leah and Rachel.

Lach, Lachlan: (Gaelic) "fjord; fjordland."

Lacy: (Latin) "from Latius; estate."

Ladd: (Middle English) "attendant."

Laibrook: (Old English) "path by the brook."

Laidley: (Old English) "from the watercourse meadow."

Laird: (Celtic) "proprietor."

Lake: the English word used as a first name.

Lamar: (Old German) "land famous." Lamar Alexander, governor of Tennessee.

Lambert: (Teutonic) "rich in land."
Also: **Bert, Lamberto (Sp).**

Lamont: (Scandinavian) "a lawyer."
Also: **Lamond.**

Lance: (Anglo-Saxon) "spear."

Also: **Lancelot, Lancey, Launce, Launcelot.**

Lander: (Middle English) "owner of a grassy plain." Also: **Landers.**

Landon: (Anglo-Saxon) "from the long hill." Also: **Langdon, Langston.**

Lane: (Anglo-Saxon) "from the country road." Also: **Layne.**

Lanford: see Langford. Lanford Wilson, playwright.

Lang: (Teutonic) "tall."

Langdon: see Landon.

Langford: (Old English) "dweller at the long ford." Also: **Lanford.**

Langley: (Old English) "from the long meadow."

Langston: (Old English) "tall man's town." See also Landon.

Langworth: (Old English) "from the long enclosure."

Lark: (Middle English) the songbird celebrated for its beautiful song during flight.

Larkin: variant of Lawrence.

Larry: see Lawrence.

Lars, Larz: see Lawrence. Lar Lubovitch, choreographer.

Larson: (Scandinavian) "son of Lars."

Latham: (Old Norse) "from the barns."

Lathrop: (Anglo-Saxon) "of the village." Also: **Lathrope.**

Latimer: (Anglo-Saxon) "Latin master or teacher."

Launcelot: see Lance.

Lauren, Laurence, Laurent, Laurindo: see Lawrence. Laurindo Almeida, jazz guitarist.

Lawford: (Old English) "from the ford at the hill."

Lawler: (Irish Gaelic) "mumbler."

Lawley: (Old English) "from the hill meadow."

Lawrence: (Latin) "laurel; crowned with laurel." Sir Laurence Olivier, actor. Also: **Larkin, Larry, Lars (Scand), Larz, Lauren, Laurence, Laurent (Fr), Laurie, Loren, Lorenz (Ger), Lorenzo (It, Sp), Lori, Lorin, Lorry, Lowrie.**

Lawson: (Old English) "son of Lawrence." Lawson Inada, poet.

Lawton: (Old English) "man of refinement." Also: **Laughton.**

Layton: see Leighton.

Lazarus: see Eleazer. Lazarus Sims, basketball player.

Lea: see Lee.

Leal: (Middle English) "loyal."

Leander: (Greek) "lion-man; brave." Leander Wapshot, New England hero of John Cheever's humorous novel *The Wapshot Chronicle* (1957). Also: **Leandro (It, Sp), Lee.**

Leandro: see Leander.

Lear: (Teutonic) "of the meadow." The aged monarch of Shakespeare's *King Lear.*

Lee: (Anglo-Saxon) "meadow; sheltered."
Also: **Lea, Leigh.** Also used as diminutive of Ashley, Leander, Leo and Leopold.

Leggett: (Old French) "envoy or delegate."

Leicester: *see* Lester.

Leif: (Old Norse) "beloved one." Leif Eriksson, explorer.

Leigh: *see* Lee. Leigh Donovan, cyclist.

Leighton: (Old English) "dweller at the meadow farm."
Also: **Layton, Leyton.**

Leith: (Scotch Gaelic) "wide river."

Leland: (Anglo-Saxon) "of the lowlands." Leland Stanford, businessman, politician.
Also: **Lealand, Leeland.**

Lemuel: (Hebrew) "consecrated to God." Lemuel Gulliver, of Jonathan Swift's *Gulliver's Travels* (1726). Lem Barney, football player.

Len, Lennie, Lenny: forms of Leo/Leonard.

Lennon: (Irish Gaelic) "little cloak."

Lennox: (Scotch Gaelic) "elm-tree grove."

Leo: (Latin) "lion." Leo is the 5th constellation of the Zodiac.
Also: **Leon, Lionel, Lyon.** *See also* Leonard, Leopold.

Leonard: (Teutonic) "brave as a lion." Leonard Bernstein, composer, conductor; Leonardo DiCaprio, actor.

Also: **Leonidas, Leonide, Len, Lennard, Lennie, Lenny.**

Leopold: (Teutonic) "brave for the people; patriotic." Leopold Stokowski, conductor.
Also: **Lee, Leo.**

Leroy: *see* Elroy.

Les: short form of Leslie, Lester.

Leslie: (Celtic) "from the gray fort."
Also: **Les, Lesley.**

Lester: (Anglo-Saxon) "from the army; camp." Lester Young, jazz musician.
Also: **Leicester, Les.**

LeVar: (French) "a bear." LeVar Burton, actor.

Leverett: (Old French) "young rabbit."

Leverton: (Old English) "from the rush farm."

Levi: (Hebrew) "united." Biblical: Jacob's son by Leah.
Also: **Levy.**

Lewis: (Teutonic) "renowned in battle." Lewis Thomas, physician, author.
Also: **Aloysius, Clovis, Lew, Lewes, Lou, Louie, Louis, Ludovick, Ludvig, Ludwig (Ger), Luigi (It), Luis (Sp).**

Liam: (Gaelic) an Irish form of William. Liam Neeson, actor.

Lincoln: (Celtic) "from the place by the pool; riverbank." Lincoln Steffens, journalist.
Also: **Linc, Link.**

Lind: (Old English) "dweller at the lime tree."

Lindberg: (Old German) "linden-tree hill."
Also: **Lindbergh.**

Lindell: (Old English) "dweller at the linden-tree valley."

Lindley: (Old English) "at the linden-tree meadow."

Lindon: see Lyndon.

Lindsay, Lindsey: (Old English) "pool island." Lindsay Anderson, film director.

Linford: (Old English) "from the linden-tree ford."

Link: (Old English) "from the bank." See also Lincoln.

Linley: (Old English) "from the flax enclosure."

Linn: see Lynn.

Linus: (Hebrew) "flaxen-haired." Linus Pauling, Nobel prize–winning chemist.

Lionel: see Leo. Lionel Hampton, jazz musician.

Lisandro: (Greek) "liberator of men."
Also: **Lysandros.**

Litton: (Old English) "hillside town."

Livingston: (Old English) "from Leif's town." Livingston Taylor, pop musician.

Llewellyn: (Welsh) "lionlike."
Also: **Lielo, Llew, Lyn.**

Lloyd: (Welsh) "gray; dark." Andrew Lloyd Webber, theatrical composer.

Locke: (Old English) "dweller in the stronghold."

Lockhart: (Scottish) "a small enclosure."

Logan: (Scotch Gaelic) "little hollow."

Lombard: (Latin) "long-bearded one."

Lon, Lonny: see Alphonse, Zebulon.

Longfellow: (English/French) "tall companion." Longfellow Deeds, hero portrayed by Gary Cooper in Frank Capra film *Mr. Deeds Goes to Town.*

Lorcan: (Gaelic) "little fierce one."

Loren, Lorenz, Lorenzo, Lorry: see Lawrence, Loring. Lorenz Hart, lyricist (1895–1943).
Also: **Lorin.**

Lorimer: (Latin) "lover of horses."

Loring: (Teutonic) from Lorraine.
Also: **Loredo, Loren, Lorry.**

Lorne: a Scottish place name.

Lothar: see Luther.

Lou, Louis: see Lewis.

Lovett: (Teutonic) "little wolf."

Lowell: (Anglo-Saxon) "beloved." Lowell Thomas, radio commentator.
Also: **Lovel, Lovell.**

Lowrie: see Lawrence.

Loyal: (Old French) "true, faithful." Loy Vaught, basketball player.
Also: **Loyall.**

Lucano: (Latin) "light."
Also: **Lucio.**

Lucas: see Lucius.

Lucien: (French) "light."
Also: **Jean-Luc, Luc, Lucin.**

Lucius: (Latin) "light." Luciano Pavarotti, opera singer.
Also: **Luca, Lucas, Luce, Lucian, Luciano (It), Lukasz (Pol), Luke, Lukev.**

Ludlow: (Old English) "dweller at the prince's hill."

Ludovick, Ludvig: see Lewis.

Luigi: Italian form of Lewis.

Luis: Spanish form of Lewis. Luis Alvarez, physicist.

Luke: see Lucius. Biblical: companion of Paul and author of the third Gospel and Acts.
Also: **Lucky.**

Lundy: (French) "born on Monday."

Lunn: (Irish Gaelic) "strong, fierce."

Lunt: (Old Norse) "from the grove."

Lutero: a Spanish form of Luther.

Luther: (Teutonic) "renowned warrior." Luther Burbank, botanist; Luther Vandross, soul singer.
Also: **Lothair, Lothar, Lothario, Lutero (Sp).**

Lyle: (French) "from the island." Lyle Lovett, country singer.
Also: **Lisle, Lyell.**

Lyman: (Old English) "man of the plains." Lyman Beecher, religious leader, father of Harriet Beecher Stowe.

Lyndon: (Old English) "hill with lime trees." Lyndon B. Johnson, 36th U.S. President.
Also: **Lindon.**

Lynn: (Anglo-Saxon) "from the waterfalls." Lynn Swann, football player, announcer.
Also: **Linn.**

Lyon: see Leo.

Lysander: (Greek) "liberator."
Also: **Sandy.**

Lytton: (English) "village on a roaring stream." Lytton Strachey, British writer.

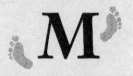

Mac: (Celtic) "the son of." Diminutive for any name beginning with Mac- or Mc-.
Also: **Mack.**

MacAdam: (Scotch Gaelic) "son of Adam."

Macaulay: (Celtic) "son of the rock." Macaulay Culkin, actor.

MacDonald: (Scotch Gaelic) "son of Donald."

Macedonio: (Greek) from Macedonia.

Mackenzie: (Scottish) "son of Kenzie." Sir Mackenzie Bowell, Canadian prime minister.
Also: **McKenzie.**

MacKinley: (Irish Gaelic) "skillful leader." MacKinlay Kantor, Pulitzer prize–winning novelist.

biblical: the
chael.
Michal (Pol),
ick, Mickey,
Mike, Mischa
h, Mitchell.

ish form of Mi-

ican Indian) "rac-

in) from Milan. Mi-
era, Czech author
Unbearable Lightness

atin) "soldier." Miles
jazz musician.
ilo, Myles.

: (Old English)
ller at the mill ford."

d: (Old English) "a mil-
Millard Fillmore, 13th
President.

urn: (Old English) "of
stream by the mill."

er: (Middle English)
grain-grinder."
lso: Millar, Mills.

ilne: (Old English) "a mill."
A. A. Milne, author of Win-
nie-the-Pooh.

ilo: (Latin) "miller." See
also Miles.

Milton: (Anglo-Saxon) "from
the mill town." Name originally associated with the
poet John Milton. Milton
Berle, "Mr. Television."
Also: **Milt.**

Milward: (Old English) "mill
keeper."

Min: (Chinese) "the people;
sharp, keen." Traditionally

combined with a second
name.

Miner: (Old French) "a
miner."

Mischa: (Hebrew) "Who is
like God?" Mischa Elman,
violinist. See also Michael.

Mitchell: variant of Michael.
Also: **Mitch.**

Moana: (Hawaiian) "the open
sea."

Modesto: (Spanish) "modest."

Modred: (Old English) "courageous counselor." The
treacherous nephew of King
Arthur in the legend.

Mohammad: (Arabic) "worthy
of praise." The Prophet of
Islam.
Also: **Mohammed, Muhammad.**

Monroe: (Celtic) "from the
red swamp." Monroe Stahr,
tragic movie producer in
Fitzgerald's unfinished novel
The Last Tycoon.
Also: **Munro.**

Montague: (Latin) "from the
pointed mountain."
Also: **Montagu, Monte.**

Montana: (Latin) "mountain";
the name of the western
state.

Monte: see Montague, Montgomery.

Monterey: (Spanish) "mountain king"; a place name.

Montgomery: (French)
"mountain hunter"; a
French place name.
Also: **Monte, Monty.**

Monty: see Montague, Montgomery.

McLean: (Scottish) "son of the
servant of St. John." McLean
Stevenson, actor.

MacMurray: (Irish Gaelic)
"son of the mariner."
Also: **Murray.**

Macnair: (Gaelic) "son of the
heir."

Macy: (Old French) "from
Matthew's estate."

Maddock: (Celtic) "fire; beneficent."
Also: **Maddox, Madoc.**

Maden: see Matthew.

Madison: (Teutonic) "mighty
in battle." James Madison,
4th U.S. President.
Also: **Maddie.**

Magee: (Irish Gaelic) "son of
the fiery one."

Magnus: (Latin) "great one."

Maitland: (Old English)
"dweller at the meadow-
land."

Major: the military title used
as a first name.

Malachi: (Hebrew) "my messenger." Biblical: the pro-
phetic Book of Malachi.
Also: **Malachy.**

Malcolm: (Celtic) "dove."
Malcolm Forbes, business-
man.

Malik: (Arabic) "king."
Also: **Maliki.**

Malin: (Old English) "little
war-mighty one."

Mallory: (Latin) "luckless."

Maloney: (Irish Gaelic) "devoted to Sunday worship."

Malvin: (Celtic) "chief."

Mandel: (German) "almond."
Mandy Patinkin, actor.

Manfred: (Old English)
"peaceful man." Literary:
the lonely hero of Lord Byron's Manfred (1817).

Manley: (Anglo-Saxon) "the
hero's meadow." Manley
Carter, U.S. astronaut.

Manning: (Old English) "son
of the hero."

Manny, Manuel: see Emmanuel.

Mansfield: (Old English)
"from the field by the small
river."

Manton: (Old English) "from
the hero's estate."

Manuel: see Emmanuel. Manuel Puig, novelist.

Manville: (Old French) "from
the great estate."

Marc: French form of Mark.

Marcel: French form of Mark.
Marcel Proust, French
writer.

Marcello: Italian form of
Mark. Marcello Mastroianni,
Italian actor.

March: see Mark.

Marcos: see Mark.

Marcus: see Mark.

Marden: (Old English) "from
the pool valley."

Mariner: (Latin) "of the sea."
Marriner Stoddard Eccles,
American banker, econo-
mist.
Also: **Marino.**

Mario: (Latin) "martial one."
Also: **Marius.**

Mark: (Latin) "belonging to Mars; a warrior." Biblical: author of the second of the Gospels.
Also: **Marc, Marcel (Fr), Marcello (It), March, Marcos (Sp), Marcus, Marcy, Marek, Mars.** See also Martin.

Marland: (Old English) "from the lake land."

Marlon: a form of Merlin. Marlon Brando, actor.
Also: **Marlen, Marlin.**

Marley: (Old English) "from the lake meadow."

Marlow: (Old English) "from the hill by the lake."
Also: **Marlowe.**

Marmaduke: (Celtic) "sea leader."
Also: **Duke.**

Marmion: (Old French) "very small one."

Maron: (Arabic) "male saint."

Marsden: (Anglo-Saxon) "from the marsh valley." Marsden Hartley, painter.
Also: **Denny.**

Marsh: (Old English) "from the marsh."

Marshall: (French) "farrier; caretaker of horses." Marshall McLuhan, media theorist.
Also: **Marsh, Marshal.**

Marston: see Marsden.

Marten: see Martin.

Martin: (Latin) a form of Mark; "warlike." St. Martin of Tours.
Also: **Marten, Martino, Marty.**

Marty: short form of Martin.

Marvin: see Irvin.

Marwood: (Old English) "from the lake forest."

Maslin: (Old French) "little Thomas."
Also: **Maslen, Maslon.**

Mason: (Latin) "stoneworker."

Mather: (Old English) "powerful army."

Mathias: see Matthew.

Matthew: (Hebrew) "God's gift." Biblical: One of the 12 disciples and author of the first Gospel.
Also: **Maddis, Maden, Mat, Mateo (Sp) Mathias, Matt, Matteo (It), Matthias, Matty.**

Maurice: (Latin) "dark; Moorish." Maurice Sendak, children's book author, illustrator.
Also: **Maurey, Mauricio (Sp), Maury, Merrick, Morel, Morice, Morris, Morry, Morse, Murray, Seymour.**

Mauricio: a Spanish form of Maurice.

Maury: a form of Maurice. Maury Povich, television personality.

Max: short form of Maximillian, Maxwell. Also given as an independent name.

Maxfield: (English) "Mack's field." Maxfield Parrish, artist, illustrator (1870–1966).

Maxime: (Latin) "the greatest." Maxime Du Camp, French writer and photographer.
Also: **Maximo.**

Maximillian: (Latin) "the greatest."

Also: **Max, Maxey, Maxie, Maxim, Maximo (Sp).** See also Max, Maxime.

Maxwell: (Anglo-Saxon) "Mack's well." Maxwell Perkins, book editor.
Also: **Max.**

Mayer: (Latin) "greater one."

Mayfield: (Old English) "from the warrior's field."

Mayhew: (Old French) "gift of Jehovah."

Maynard: (Anglo-Saxon) "mightily strong." Maynard Ferguson, jazz musician.

Mayo: (Irish Gaelic) "from the plain of the yew trees."

Mead: (Old English) "from the meadow." Meade Lux Lewis, jazz musician.

Medwin: (Teutonic) "strong friend."
Also: **Winnie.**

Mel: short form of names beginning Mel-. Also used as an independent name. Mel Tormé, singer.

Melbourne: (Old English) "from the millstream"; the Australian city.

Meldon: (Old English) "dweller at the mill hill."

Meldrick: (Old English) "powerful mill." Meldrick Taylor, Olympic boxer.

Mellor: (Teutonic) "miller."

Melville, Melvil: (French) "a place." Melvil Dewey, inventor of the Dewey decimal system (1876).
Also: **Mel.**

Micah: a form of Michael. Biblical: prophet.

Michael: (Hebrew) "Who is

like God?" B
archangel M
Also: **Micael,**
Michel (Fr),
Miguel (Sp),
(Slavic), Mit

Miguel: Spa
chael.

Mika: (Ame
coon."

Milan: (La
Ian Kund
of The
of Bein

Miles: (L
Davis,
Also: M

Milford
"dwe

Millar
ler.
U.S

Merle: (Ang
nature
blackbi
country
Also: **Merl**

Merlin: (Ang
falcon." M
ball player.
Also: **Marl, Ma**
Marlon, Merl, N

Merrick: see Ma

Merrill: see Myroi

Merritt: (Anglo-Sax
merit."

Merton: (Anglo-Saxon
the place by the sea.

Mervin, Merwin: see Irv
Mervyn LeRoy, film dir
(1900–1987).

Mesa: the Spanish word for
"table" describes a flat, tablelike mountain or piece of land.

Meyer: (Teutonic) "farmer." Meyer Guggenheim, industrialist.
Also: **Mayer.**

Moore: (Old French) "dark-complexioned."

Morcant: *see* Morgan.

Mordecai: (Hebrew) "a wise counselor." Biblical: in the Book of Esther, his sage advice ensured the survival of his people.

Morel, Morrell: (Latin) "swarthy."

Moreland: (Old English) "from the moorland."

Morgan: (Celtic) "from the sea; sea white." Morgan Freeman, actor.
Also: **Morcant.**

Morley: (Anglo-Saxon) "from the moor meadow." Morley Safer, broadcast journalist.
Also: **Morely.**

Morris: *see* Maurice.

Morrison: (Old English) "son of Maurice."
Also: **Morrissey.**

Morse: *see* Maurice.

Mortimer: (Latin) "from the quiet water." Mortimer Adler, American philosopher.
Also: **Mort, Mortie, Morty.**

Morven: (Irish Gaelic) "great mountain peak."

Moses: (Egyptian) "savior." Biblical: liberator of Israel. Mose Allison, jazz singer.
Also: **Moe, Mose, Moss.**

Moss: *see* Moses.

Mostyn: (Welsh) "field-fortress."

Muhammad: (Arabic) "worthy of praise." The Prophet of Islam.
Also: **Mohammad, Mohammed.**

Muir: (Celtic) "moor."

Mulgrew: the surname used as a first name. Mulgrew Miller, jazz artist.

Munro: *see* Monroe. Munro Leaf, children's author, illustrator.

Murdoch: (Celtic) "prosperous from the sea."
Also: **Murdock, Murtagh.**

Murphy: (Irish Gaelic) "sea warrior."

Murray: (Celtic) "settlement by the sea."
Also: **Murrey, Murry.** *See also* Maurice.

Myles: *see* Miles.

Myron: (Greek) "fragrant." Myron Goldsmith, architect.
Also: **Merrill.**

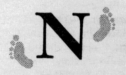

Naaman: "agreeable." Biblical: the Aramaean general cured by Elisha.

Nahum: *see* Naum.

Nairn: (Scotch Gaelic) "dweller at the alder-tree river"; a county in northeastern Scotland.

Naldo: (Teutonic) "power"; a Spanish contraction of Ronald.

Napoleon: (German) "obscure." Nappy Brown, rhythm-and-blues singer; Nap Lajoie, baseball player.

Narcissus: (Greek) "daffodil." Mythology: the Greek youth who fell in love with his own reflection.

Nash: (English) "the ash trees."

Nate: *see* Nathaniel.

Nathan: *see* Nathaniel.
Also: **Nat.**

Nathaniel: (Hebrew) "gift of God." Biblical: one of the disciples of Jesus.
Also: **Nat, Nate, Nathan, Nathanael, Natie, Natty.**

Naum: (Hebrew) "comforter." Biblical: Old Testament prophet. Naum Gabo, sculptor.

Navarro: (Spanish) "plains."

Naylor: (Teutonic) "one who fastens or secures with nails."

Nazareth: (Hebrew) from Nazareth.

Neal: (Celtic) "champion." Neil Armstrong, first astronaut to step on the moon.
Also: **Neale, Nealey, Neil, Nels, Niall (Irish), Niles.** *See also* Cornelius.

Nealon: *see* Neal.

Ned: short form of Edmund, Edward, Norton. Also given as an independent name.

Nehemiah: (Hebrew) "God is comfort." Biblical: Old Testament prophet.

Nehsa: (Egyptian) "a watcher."

Neil: *see* Neal.

Nels: a Scandinavian form of Neil.

Nelson: (Celtic) "son of Neal/Neil." Nelson Rockefeller, governor and vice president.
Also: **Neilson.** *See also* Cornelius.

Nemo: (Greek) "from the glen."

Neriah: (Hebrew) "God lights thy pathway."
Also: **Neri.**

Nero: (Italian) "black; dark."

Nestor: (Greek) "venerable wisdom." In Greek mythology, king of Pylos. Nestor Almendros, cinematographer.
Also: **Nessie, Nessim.**

Netra: (Sanskrit) "a leader."

Nevada: (Spanish) "snowy"; the Western state. Nevada Smith, of the film and TV series of the same name.

Neville: (Latin) "from the new town." Neville Brand, actor; Neville Chamberlain, British prime minister.
Also: **Nev, Nevil.**

Nevin: (Anglo-Saxon) "nephew."
Also: **Nevins, Niven.**

Newel, Newell: *see* Noel.

Newland: (Old English) "dweller on reclaimed land."
Also: **Niland.**

Newlin: (Old Welsh) "dweller at the new pool."

Newman: the surname used as a first name.

Newton: (Anglo-Saxon) "from the new estate."
Also: **Newt.**

Newt: *see* Newton.

Niall: an Irish form of Neal.

Nicholas: (Greek) "victory of the people." St. Nicholas, patron saint of Russia and of children.
Also: **Claus, Klaus, Nichol, Nicholl, Nick, Nicky, Nicol, Nicolas (Fr, Sp).**

Nick: *see* Nicholas.

Nico: a form of Nicodemus.

Nicodemus: (Greek) "the people's conqueror."
Also: **Nick, Nicky.**

Nicol: *see* Nicholas. Nicol Williamson, actor.

Nigel: (Latin) "dark; black." Nigel Bruce, actor.

Nils: a Scandinavian form of Neil. Niels Bohr, Danish physicist and pioneer in atomic theory.

Niles: *see* Neal.

Nino: (Spanish) "little boy."

Nixon: (Old English) "son of Nicholas."

Noah: (Hebrew) "rest; comfort; peace." Biblical: hero of the flood story. Noah Webster, compiler of the standard dictionary.
Also: **Noadiah, Noe.**

Noam: (Hebrew) "sweetness, friendship." Noam Chomsky, author.

Noble: (Latin) "renowned; noble." Noble Sissle, songwriter.
Also: **Nobel.**

Nobu: (NOH-boo) (Japanese) "believe."

Noe: (Hebrew) "rest." Noe Munoz, baseball player.

Noel: (Latin) "Christmas."
Also: **Newel, Newell, Noelle, Nowell.**

Nolan: (Celtic) "famous."
Also: **Noland.**

Noll: *see* Oliver.

Norbert: (Teutonic) "sea brightness." Norbert Wu, photographer.
Also: **Bert.**

Norman: (Teutonic) "man from the North; of Normandy."
Also: **Norm, Normand, Normie, Norris.**

Norris: *see* Norman.

North: (Old English) "man from the North."

Northcliff: (Old English) "from the north cliff."

Northrop: (Old English) "from the north farm."
Also: **Northrup.**

Norton: (Anglo-Saxon) "from the north place."
Also: **Ned, Norty.**

Norval, Norvald: *see* Norville.

Norvel: *see* Norville.

Norville: (Old Anglo-French) "from the north estate."
Also: **Norval, Norvel, Norvil.**

Norvin: (Teutonic) "man from the North."

Norward: (Teutonic) "the guard at the northern gate."
Also: **Norwood, Norword.**

Noton: (American Indian) "the wind."

Nowell: a form of Noel.

Nunzio: (Italian) "messenger."

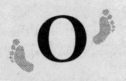

Oakes: (Middle English) "dweller at the oak trees."

Oakley: (Anglo-Saxon) "from the oak-tree meadow."

Obadiah: (Hebrew) "the Lord's servant." Biblical: the Book of Obadiah.
Also: **Obe, Obediah.**

Obert: (Old German) "wealthy, brilliant one."

Ocean: the word used as a first name.

Octavius: (Latin) "eighth." Octavio Paz, Mexican poet.
Also: **Octave, Octavian, Octavio, Octavus, Tavey.**

Odell: (Teutonic) "wealthy."
Also: **Odin, Odo.**

Odolf: (Old German) "wealthy wolf."

Odoric: (Latin) "son of a good man."

Ogden: (Anglo-Saxon) "from the oak valley." Ogden Nash, poet.

Ogilvie: (Pictish-Scotch) "from the high peak."

Oglesby: (Old English) "awe-inspiring."

Olaf: (Scandinavian) "ancestor." Olaf II, king and patron saint of Norway.
Also: **Olav, Ole, Olen, Oley, Olle, Olof.**

Ole: pet form of Olaf.

Oleg: (Russian) "holy." Oleg Cassini, fashion designer.

Olin: see Olaf. Olin Browne, golfer.

Oliver: (Latin) "olive; peace." Oliver Wendell Holmes, Jr., Supreme Court justice.
Also: **Oliverio (Sp), Olivier (Fr), Ollie, Noll, Nollie, Nolly.**

Ollie: pet form of Oliver.

Olney: (Old English) "Olla's island."

Omar: (Arabic) "who has a long life." Omar Bradley, U.S. general; Omar Sharif, actor.

O'Neal: (Celtic) "of the champion's line."
Also: **O'Neil, O'Neill.**

Onslow: (Old English) "zealous one's hill."

Oral, Orel: (Latin) "endowed with speech." Orel Hershiser, baseball pitcher.

Oram: (Old English) "from the riverbank enclosure."

Ordway: (Anglo-Saxon) "spear fighter."

Oren: (Hebrew) "pine." Oren Arnold, children's author.
Also: **Orin, Orrin.**

Orford: (Old English) "dweller at the cattle ford."

Oriel, Oriole: see Aurelio.

Orion: (Latin) "giant." Mythology: the famed hunter.

Orlando: Italian form of Roland. Orlando Cepeda, baseball player.
Also: **Orland.**

Orlin: (Greek) "golden radiance."
Also: **Orleans, Orley.**

Ormond: (Irish) "red."
Also: **Orman, Ormand.**

Oro: (Spanish) "golden one."

Orrick: (Old English) "dweller at the ancient oak tree."

Orson: (Latin) "bear." Orson Welles, filmmaker.
Also: **Orsini, Orsino.**

Orton: (Old English) "from the shore farmstead."

Orval: (Old English) "spear-mighty."

Orville: (French) "lord of the manor." Orville Wright, aviation pioneer.
Also: **Orvil.**

Orvin: (Old English) "spear friend."

Osbert: (Anglo-Saxon) "divinely bright."
Also: **Bert, Bertie, Berty, Oz, Ozzie.**

Osborn: (Anglo-Saxon) "divinely strong." Osborn Elliot, journalist.
Also: **Osborne, Osbourne, Osburn.**

Oscar: (Anglo-Saxon) "divine spear." Oscar Arias Sanchez, president of Costa Rica, winner of the Nobel Peace Prize.
Also: **Os, Oskar (Pol), Ozzie.**

Osgood: (Teutonic) "gift of our Lord."

Osmar: (Old English) "divinely glorious."

Osmond: (Teutonic) "he is protected by God."
Also: **Osman, Osmund, Ozzie.**

Osred: (Old English) "divine counselor."

Osric: (Old English) "divine ruler."

Ossian: "fawn." Mythology: the son of Finn.
Also: **Oisin, Ossin.**

Ossie: familiar form of names beginning Os-. Ossie Davis, actor.

Oswald: (Anglo-Saxon) "divine power."
Also: **Os, Oz.**

Othman: (Old German) "prosperous man."

Otis: variant of Otto. Otis Chandler, newspaper publisher.
Also: **Ottis.**

Otto: (Teutonic) "wealthy; prosperous." Otto Preminger, film director.

Owen: (Welsh) "wellborn." Owen Wister, writer.
Also: **Owain (Welsh).**

Oxford: (Old English) "from the oxen ford."

Oxton: (Old English) "from the ox enclosure."

Ozias: Greek form of Uzziah.

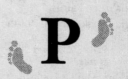

P

Pablo: Spanish form of Paul. Pablo Casals, cellist.

Pacifico: (Latin) "quiet, peaceful."

Paco: Spanish form of Frank.

Paddy: see Patrick.

Padgett: (French) "young attendant."
Also: **Paget.**

Padma: (Sanskrit) "the lotus flower"; the Padma River in India.

Page: (French) "servant to the royal court." Page Smith, historian.
Also: **Paige.**

Paget: see Padgett.

Paine: (Latin) "countryman; rustic; pagan." Payne Stewart, golfer.
Also: **Payne.**

Paley: see Paul.

Palmer: (Latin) "the palm-bearer; pilgrim."

Pano: (Hawaiian) "deep blue-black, as in the ocean depths."

Paolo: Italian form of Paul.

Paris: in contemporary usage, the French place name used as a first name. In Greek mythology, the handsome prince whose abduction of Helen caused the Trojan War.

Parish: see Parrish.

Park: (Anglo-Saxon) "of the park."
Also: **Parke. (Chinese) "the cypress tree."**

Parker: (Middle English) "park keeper." Parker Stevenson, actor.

Parkin: (Old English) "little Peter."

Parle: (Old French) "little Peter."

Parnel, Parnell: see Peter.

Parrish: (Old English) "an ecclesiastical district."
Also: **Parish.**

Parry: (French) "guardian; protector."

Pascal: (French) "born at Easter."
Also: **Pasquale (It).**

Pate: (Gaelic) "noble."

Patrick: (Latin) "noble; patrician." St. Patrick, patron saint of Ireland.
Also: **Paddy, Padraic, Pat, Pate, Patric, Rick.**

Patton: (Old English) "from the combatant's estate."
Also: **Pat, Paton.**

Paul: (Latin) "little." Biblical: St. Paul the Apostle.
Also: **Pablo (Sp), Paley, Paolo (It), Paulie, Pawel (Pol).**

Paxton: (Teutonic) "from afar; a traveler."
Also: **Packston, Paxon.**

Payne: see Paine.

Payton: see Peyton.

Pearce: see Peter.

Pedro: Spanish form of Peter. Pedro Pablo Morales, American Olympic swimmer.

Pell: (Old English) "mantle or scarf."

Pelton: (Old English) "from the estate by the pool."

Pembroke: (Celtic) "from the headland."

Penley: (Old English) "enclosed pasture."

Penn: (Old German) "commander." Penn Jillette, of Penn & Teller, the comedy act.

Penrod: (Old German) "famous commander."

Pepin: (Old German) "petitioner."

Percival: (French) "valley-piercer." Percival Lowell, U.S. amateur astronomer who helped discover Pluto.
Also: **Parsifal, Perce, Perceval, Percy, Purcell.**

Percy: see Percival. Percy Bysshe Shelley, English poet.

Peregrine: (Latin) "traveler." Peregrine White was the first child to be born of English parents in New England. He was born on the *Mayflower* in Cape Cod Bay.
Also: **Perry, Pippin.**

Pernell: Pernell Whitaker, Olympic boxer.

Perry: (Anglo-Saxon) "pear tree." Perry Ellis, fashion designer; Perry (Pierino) Como, singer. *See also* Peregrine.

Perth: (Pictish-Celtic) "thornbush thicket."

Peter: (Greek) "rock; stone." Biblical: the nickname given by Christ to the apostle Simon: "Thou art Peter, and upon this rock I will build my church."
Also: **Parnel, Parnell, Pearce, Pedr (Welsh), Pedro (Sp), Pernel, Pernell, Perrin, Pete, Petey, Petie, Petrie, Pierce,**

Pierre (Fr), Pieter (Dutch), Pietro (It).

Petros: a form of Peter.

Peverell: (Old French) "piper."

Peyton: (Latin) "noble; patrician." Peyton Rous, American physician.

Phelan: (Celtic) "wolf; brave as a wolf."

Philbert: (Teutonic) "a radiant soul."
Also: **Filbert, Bert.**

Philip: (Greek) "lover of horses." Biblical: one of the 12 disciples.
Also: **Felipe, Flip, Phelps, Phil, Philippe, Phillip, Phillippe.**

Philo: (Greek) "love."

Phineas: (Hebrew) "oracle." P. T. (Phineas Taylor) Barnum, showman.

Pickford: (Old English) "from the ford at the peak."

Pickworth: (Old English) "from the tree cutter's estate."

Pierce: see Peter. Pierce Brosnan, actor.

Pierre: French form of Peter.

Pierson: (Greek) "son of Peter."
Also: **Pearson, Peerson, Pierce.**

Pilgrim: (Latin) "one who travels new land with some spiritual aim."

Pin: (Vietnamese) "faithful boy."

Pitney: (Old English) "preserving one's island."

Pitte: (Old English) "from the pit."
Also: **Pitt.**

Pius: (Latin) "pious."

Placido: (Spanish) "placid." Placido Domingo, opera singer.

Plato: the Greek philosopher.

Platt: (Old French) "from the flatland."

Polk: the surname used as a first name.

Pollard: (Teutonic) "cropped hair."

Pollock: (Old English) "little Paul."

Pomeroy: (Old French) "from the apple orchard."

Pontius: (Latin) "the fifth son."

Porter: (Latin) "gatekeeper." Porter Wagoner, country singer.

Potter: (English) "a potter." Potter Stewart, Supreme Court justice.

Powell: (Celtic) "alert."

Prentice: (Latin) "learner; apprentice."
Also: **Prentis.**

Prescott: (Anglo-Saxon) "of the priest's house."
Also: **Scott.**

Presley: (Old English) "dweller at the priest's meadow."

Preston: (Anglo-Saxon) "of the priest's place." Preston Sturges, film director, screenwriter (1898–1959).

Prewitt: (Old French) "little valiant one."
Also: **Pruitt.**

Primo: (Italian) "first child born to a family." Primo Carnera, boxer.

Prince: (Latin) "prince."

Prior: (Latin) "superior; head of a monastery."
Also: **Pryor.**

Priya: (Sanskrit) "beloved."

Proctor: (Latin) "leader."
Also: **Procter.**

Prosper: (Latin) "the fortunate one." Prosper Mérimée, French author.
Also: **Prospero.**

Prudent: a Puritan virtue name.

Pruitt: *see* Prewitt.

Putnam: (Anglo-Saxon) "dweller of the pond."

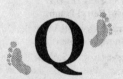

Quan: (Chinese) "authority; whole, complete." Traditionally combined with a second name.

Quartus: (Latin) "the fourth son."

Quentin: (Latin) "fifth." Quentin Tarantino, film director.
Also: **Quent, Quint, Quintin, Quinton.**

Quigley: (Irish Gaelic) "distaff."

Quillon: (Latin) "sword."
Also: **Quill.**

Quinby: (Scandinavian) "of the womb of woman."
Also: **Quimby.**

Quincy: (Latin) "from the fifth son's place." Quincy Delight Jones, Jr., composer, producer.

Quinn: (Gaelic) "wise and intelligent."

Quintin, Quinton: *see* Quentin.

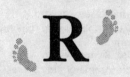

Race: *see* Horace.

Rad: a short form of names beginning Rad-.

Radbert: (Old English) "brilliant counselor."

Radburn: (Old English) "he lives by the red brook."
Also: **Radbourne, Radburne.**

Radcliffe: (Anglo-Saxon) "from the red cliff." Radcliffe Bailey, Jr., artist.
Also: **Cliff, Radcliffye.**

Radford: (Old English) "from the red ford."

Radnor: (Old English) "at the red shore." Radney Foster, country singer.

Radolf: (Old English) "wolf counselor."

Rafael: *see* Raphael.
Also: **Rafal (Polish).**

Rafer: variant of Rafael. Rafer Johnson, decathlete.

Rafferty: (Irish Gaelic) "prosperous and rich."
Also: **Rafe.**

Rafi: (Arabic) "exalted."

Rainer: (German) "strong counselor." Rainer Werner Fassbinder, film director (1946–1982).
Also: **Raine, Raines, Rainier, Ranier, Reiner.**

Raleigh: (Old English) "of the deer field."

Ralph: (Anglo-Saxon) "wolf counselor."
Also: **Ralf, Ralphie, Raoul (Fr), Raul (Sp).**

Ralston: English place name.
Also: **Ralfston, Roliston.**

Rama: (Sanskrit) "joy-bringer." The hero of Hindu lore.

Ramah: (Latin) "branch." (Hebrew) "a high place."

Rambert: (Old German) "mighty; brilliant."

Ramey: *see* Remy.

Ramon: Spanish form of Raymond.

Ramsden: (Old English) "from the ram's island."

Ramsey: (Teutonic) "raven's island." Ramsey Lewis, jazz artist.
Also: **Ramsay.**

Rana: (Sanskrit) "of royalty."

Rance: a short form of Ransom, Ranson.

Randall: *see* Randolph.

Randolph: (Anglo-Saxon) "wolf counselor."

Also: **Ralf, Ralph, Rand, Randal, Randall, Randy, Rolf, Rolfe, Rolph.**

Ranger: (Old French) "forest keeper."

Ranier: see Rainer.

Rankin: (Old English) "little shield."

Ransford: (Old English) "from the raven's ford."

Ransley: (Old English) "from the raven's meadow."

Ransom: see Ranson.
Also: **Rance, Ransome.**

Ranson: (Old English) "son of the shield." Ranson Olds, auto manufacturer.
Also: **Rance.**

Raoul: French form of Ralph. Raoul Walsh, film director (1887–1980).

Raphael: (Hebrew) "healed by God." The archangel, patron of doctors and travelers.
Also: **Rafael, Raff, Raffaello.**

Rashad: see Rashid.

Rashid, Raashid: (Arabic) "righteous counselor." Raashid Wallace, basketball player.
Also: **Rashad, Rasheed.**

Rasmus, Rastus: see Erastus.

Raul: Spanish form of Ralph. Raul Julia, actor.

Raven: (English) a bird name. Mythology: a recurring hero in mythology of Indian tribes of the Pacific Northwest coast.

Ravi: (Sanskrit) "sun." The Hindu god of the sun. Ravi Shankar, musician.

Rawling: (Old Anglo-French) "son of the wolf counselor."
Also: **Rawson.**

Rawson: (Old English) see Rawling.

Ray: familiar form of Raymond and names beginning Ra-.

Rayburn: (Old English) "of the deer's brook."

Raymond: (Teutonic) "wise protection." Raymond Chandler, writer.
Also: **Ramon, Ray, Raymund.**
See also Reginald.

Raynard: see Reynard.

Raynor: (Old Norse) "mighty army."
Also: **Rainer, Rayner.**

Razi: (Aramaic) "my secret."
Also: **Raz.**

Reade: (Anglo-Saxon) "red-haired."
Also: **Read, Reed, Reid.**

Reading: (Old English) "son of the red-haired one."
Also: **Redding.**

Reave: see Reeve.

Red: short form of names beginning Red-. Also given as an independent name. Red Grooms, artist.

Redding: see Reading.

Redford: (Old English) "from the red ford."

Redley: (Old English) "dweller at the red meadow."
Also: **Radley.**

Redmond: (Teutonic) "adviser; protector."

Redwald: (Old English) "mighty counsel."

Reece: (Old Welsh) "ardent one."
Also: **Rees, Reese, Rhett, Rhys.**

Reed: (Old English) "red-haired." Reid Cornelius, baseball player.
Also: **Reade, Reid.**

Reeve: (Middle English) "fiscal officer of a shire or county."
Also: **Reave.**

Regan: (Celtic) "royal; king."

Reginald: (Teutonic) "mighty ruler." Reginald Marsh, artist.
Also: **Raymond, Reg, Reggie, Reinhold, René, Reynold, Rinaldo (It), Ronald.**

Regis: (French) "king." Regis Philbin, TV personality.

Reid: see Reade.

Reilly: see Riley.

Reinhold: see Reginald.

Remington: (Old English) "from the raven-family estate."

Remus: (Latin) "oarsman."

Remy: (French) "from Rheims."
Also: **Ramey, Remi.**

Renato: (Latin) "born again."

Renaud: (Old French) "powerful judgment."

René: (French) "reborn." René Descartes, French philosopher.

Renfred: (Old English) "mighty and peaceful."

Renfrew: (Old Welsh) "from the still river or channel." A Scottish place name.

Renny: (Irish Gaelic) "little; powerful." Renny Harlin, film director.

Renshaw: (Old English) "from the raven forest."

Renton: (Old English) "roebuck deer estate."

Reuben: (Hebrew) "Behold a son!" Biblical: Jacob's first-born son.
Also: **Reubin, Rube, Ruben, Rubin.**

Rex: (Latin) "king." Rex Harrison, actor.

Rexford: (Old English) "dweller at the king's ford."

Reynard: (Old German) "mighty; brave."
Also: **Raynard.**

Reynold: (Old English) "mighty and powerful." See also Reginald.

Reza: (Arabic) "accepting."

Rhett: see Reece. Rhett Butler, of Gone with the Wind.

Rhodes: (Middle English) "dweller at the crucifixes."

Rhys: see Reece.

Richard: (Teutonic) "powerful ruler." Richard the Lion-Hearted, king of England.
Also: **Dick, Ricardo (Sp), Rich, Richie, Rick, Rickert, Ricky, Ritchie.**

Richmond: a French place name meaning "lofty mountain."

Rick: a form of Alaric, Richard, etc., but also used as an independent name.
Also: **Ric, Rik.**

Rickward: (Old English) "powerful guardian."

Riddock: (Irish Gaelic) "from the smooth field." Riddick Bowe, boxer.

Rider: (Old English) "knight or horseman."
Also: **Ryder.**

Ridge: (Old English) "from the ridge."

Ridgeway: (Old English) "from the ridge road."

Ridgley: (Old English) "he lives by the meadow's edge."

Ridley: (Old English) "from the red meadow." Ridley Scott, film director.

Ridpath: (Old English) "dweller on the red path."

Rigby: (Old English) "ruler's valley."

Rigg: (Old English) "from the ridge."

Riley: the Irish surname used as a first name.
Also: **Reilly.**

Rinaldo: see Reginald.

Ring: (Old English) "a ring." Ring Lardner, writer.

Riordan: (Irish Gaelic) "royal poet or bard."

Ripley: (Old English) "dweller at the shouter's meadow." Rip Van Winkle, sleepy protagonist of Washington Irving story (1819).

Risley: (Old English) "from the brushwood meadow."

Riston: (Old English) "from the brushwood estate."

Ritter: (North German) "a knight."

River: the English word used as a first name. River Phoenix, actor.

Roald: (Old English) "famous ruler." Roald Dahl, children's book author.

Roan: (North English) "dweller at the rowan tree."

Roarke: (Irish Gaelic) "famous ruler."
Also: **Rourke.**

Robert: (Teutonic) "of bright, shining fame."
Also: **Bob, Bobbie, Bobby, Rab, Rob, Robbie, Robby, Roberto (It, Sp), Robin, Robyn, Rupert.**

Robin, Robyn: variant of Robert; a bird's name. Robin Williams, actor; Robben Ford, musician.

Robinson: (Old English) "shining with fame." Robinson Jeffers, poet.

Rochester: (Old English) "rocky fortress."

Rock: (Old English) "from the rock." Rock Hudson, actor.

Rockley: (Old English) "from the rocky meadow."

Rockwell: (Old English) "from the rocky spring." Rockwell Kent, painter.

Rod, Roddy: short forms of Roderick, Rodney.

Roderick: (Teutonic) "renowned ruler."
Also: **Broderick, Rod, Roddy, Roderic, Rodrick, Rory.**

Rodmann: (Teutonic) "redhead."
Also: **Rod, Roddy, Rodman.**

Rodney: (Teutonic) "renowned." Rod Carew, baseball player.
Also: **Rod, Roddie, Roddy, Rodi.**

Rodwell: (Old English) "dweller at the Christian spring."

Roger: (Teutonic) "renowned spearman; famous warrior."
Also: **Dodge, Hodge, Hodgekin, Rodge.**

Roland: (Teutonic) "fame of the land." Roland Matthes, German Olympic swimmer.
Also: **Orlando (It), Rolando (Sp), Roley, Rollin, Rollo, Rowland.**

Rollo: see Roland, Rudolph.

Rolph: see Randolph, Rudolph.
Also: **Rolf, Rolfe.**

Rolt: (Old German) "famous power."

Roman: (Latin) "man from Rome." Roman Polanski, film director.
Also: **Romaine, Romano (Sp), Romayne, Rome, Romeo, Romero.**

Romeo: (Latin) "man from Rome." Hero of Shakespeare's tragedy *Romeo and Juliet.*

Romney: (Old Welsh) "curving river."

Romulus: (Latin) "citizen of Rome."
Also: **Romulo.**

Ronald: see Reginald. Ronald Reagan, 40th U.S. President.
Also: **Renaldo (Sp).**

Ronan: (Irish Gaelic) "little seal."

Ronson: (Old English) "son of mighty power."

Roosevelt: (Dutch) "rose field." Roosevelt (Rosey) Grier, football player.

Roper: (Old English) "rope maker."

Rory: (Celtic) "ruddy; red-haired." Rory Calhoun, Western film actor.
Also: **Rorie, Rorry.** *See also* Roderick.

Roscoe: (Teutonic) "from the deer forest." Roscoe Tanner, tennis player.
Also: **Ros, Rosco, Roz.**

Roslin: (Old French) "little red-haired one."

Ross: (Teutonic) "horse." Ross McDonald, detective writer.

Roswell: (Teutonic) "mighty steed."
Also: **Ros, Roswald, Roz.**

Rowan: (Irish) "red; rowan tree." Rowan Atkinson, British comedian.
Also: **Rowann, Rowe.**

Rowell: (Old English) "from the roe deer spring."

Rowley: (Old English) "dweller at the rough meadow."

Rowson: (Anglo-Irish) "son of the red-haired one."

Roxbury: (Old English) "from the rock's fortress."

Roy: (Latin) "king." *See also* Elroy.

Royal: (Old French) "regal one." Royal Ingersoll, U.S. admiral.

Royce: (French) "son of the king."

Royd: (Old Norse) "from the clearing in the forest."

Roydon: (Old English) "dweller at the rye hill."
Also: **Royden.**

Rube, Ruby: see Reuben.

Ruck: (Old English) "crow."

Rudd: (Old English) "ruddy-complexioned."

Rudolph: (Teutonic) "famed wolf." Rudolph Giuliani, New York City mayor.
Also: **Dolph, Rolfe, Rollin, Rollo, Rolph, Rudolf, Rudy.**

Rudyard: (Teutonic) "famous rod or wand." Rudyard Kipling, British novelist.

Rue: (Greek) a botanical name.

Rufus: (Latin) "red-haired." Rufus King, member of Continental Congress.
Also: **Griffin, Griffith, Rufino (Sp).**

Rugby: (Old English) "rook estate."

Rule: (Latin) "ruler."

Rumford: (Old English) "from the wide ford."

Rupert: see Robert. Rupert Murdoch, publisher.

Rush: (French) "red-haired."

Rushford: (Old English) "from the rush ford."

Ruskin: (Franco-German) "little redhead."

Russ: see Cyrus, Russell.

Russell: (Anglo-Saxon) "like a fox."
Also: **Russ, Rusel.**

Rusty: (Old French) "red-haired."

Rutherford: (Old English) "from the cattle ford." Rutherford B. Hayes, 19th U.S. President.
Also: **Rutherfurd.**

Rutland: (Old Norse) "from the root or stump land."

Rutledge: (Old English) "from the red pool."

Rutley: (Old English) "from the stump meadow."

Ryan: (Irish Gaelic) "little king."

Rycroft: (Old English) "from the rye field."

Ryder: see Rider.

Rye: (Old French) "from the riverbank."

Rylan: (Old English) "dweller at the rye land." Ry (Ryland) Cooder, singer/musician.

Ryle: (Old English) "from the rye hill."

Ryley: see Riley.

Ryman: (Old English) "rye seller."

Ryton: (Old English) "from the rye enclosure."

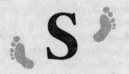

Saber: (French) "a sword."

Sabin: (Latin) "a man of the Sabine people."

Sacha: a form of the Russian name Aleksandr.

Safford: (Old English) "from the willow ford."

Sage: (English) "a wise person." Sage Moonblood, son of actor Sylvester Stallone.

Sal: see Salvador.

Salem: (Arabic) "complete, perfect peace."
Also: **Salim, Selim.**

Salisbury: (Old English) "from the guarded palace."

Salomon: (Hebrew) "peaceable; wise." Salmon P. Chase, Supreme Court chief justice.

Salton: (Old English) "from the manor-hill town."

Salvador, Salvatore: (Latin) "of the Savior"; Salvador, a Brazilian port city.
Also: **Sal, Salvidor.**

Samiir: (Arabic) "companion."

Samson: (Hebrew) "sunlike." Biblical: the hero of legendary strength.
Also: **Sam, Sammy, Sampson, Simson, Sim, Simpson.**

Samuel: (Hebrew) "name of God." Biblical: prophet who

established Saul, then David, as king of Israel.
Also: **Sam, Sammy.**

Sanborn: (Old English) "of the sandy beach."
Also: **Sanborne, Sanburn, Sandy.**

Sancho: (Spanish) "truthful; sincere."

Sanders: (Greek) "son of Alexander."
Also: **Sander, Sandor, Sandy, Saunders.** See also Alexander.

Sandy: see Alexander, Lysander, Sanborn, Sanford.

Sanford: (Old English) "by the sandy crossing." Sandy Koufax, baseball pitcher.
Also: **Sandford.**

Santana: (Spanish) "Saint Anne/Anna." Santana Dotson, football player.

Santiago: (Latin) "Saint James."

Santo: (Italian) "holy, sacred."
Also: **Santos.**

Santon: (Old English) "sandy town."

Sargent: (Latin) "a military attendant." Sargent Shriver, first director of the Peace Corps, ambassador to France.
Also: **Sarge, Sergeant.**

Sasha: a form of the Russian name Aleksandr.

Satchel: (origin uncertain). Satchel Paige, baseball player; Satchel, son of Woody Allen.

Saul: (Hebrew) "longed for; desired." Saul Bellow, Nobel prize–winning author.

Biblical: the first king of Israel.
Also: **Sol.**

Saunder, Saunders: forms of Alexander.

Saville: (North French) "willow estate."
Also: **Savill.**

Sawyer: (Celtic) "man of the woods."
Also: **Saw.**

Saxon: (Teutonic) "from a Saxon town."
Also: **Sax, Saxen.**

Sayer: (Welsh) "carpenter."
Also: **Say, Sayre.**

Scanlon: (Irish Gaelic) "a little scandal."

Schuyler: (Dutch) "a scholar; a wise man."
Also: **Sky, Skye, Skylar.**

Scott: (Latin) "a Scotsman."
Also: **Scot, Scottie, Scotty.**

Scully: (Irish Gaelic) "town crier."

Seabert: (Old English) "sea-glorious."
Also: **Seaber.**

Seaborn: (Old English) "born at sea."

Seabrook: (Old English) "from the brook by the sea."

Seamus, Shamus: Irish forms of James. Seamus Heaney, Irish poet.

Sean, Shawn: Irish forms of John. Sean Connery, actor.

Searle: (Old German) "armed one."
Also: **Searles.**

Seaton: (English) "estate by the sea."

Seaver: (English) "victorious stronghold."

Sebastian: (Greek) "respected; reverenced." St. Sebastian; Sebastian Coe, British world record holder, track and field.
Also: **Bastian, Bastien, Sebastiano (It).**

Sedgewick: (Old English) "from the village of victory."
Also: **Sedgewinn.**

Sedgley: (Old English) "from the swordsman's meadow."

Seeley: (Old English) "happy, blessed."

Seger: (Old English) "sea warrior."

Selby: (Teutonic) "from the manor farm."
Also: **Shelby.**

Selden: (Old English) "from the willow-tree valley."
Also: **Seldon.**

Selig: *see* Zelig.

Selim: (Arabic) "peaceful."
See also Salem.

Selwyn: (Teutonic) "friend at the manor." Selwyn Raab, journalist.
Also: **Wyn, Wynn.**

Seneca: (American Indian) "red paint; place of the stone." American Indian tribe.

Senior: (Old French) "lord of the manor."

Sennett: (French) "old, wise one."

Septimus: (Latin) "seventh son." Septimus Winner,

19th-century American songwriter.

Sequoia: the giant trees of California, named for the Cherokee Sequoyah, who created an alphabet for his tribe.

Serafin: (Hebrew) "ardent one."

Sereno: (Latin) "tranquil."

Serge: (Latin) "the attendant." Sergio Leone, film director; Serge Koussevitzky, conductor.
Also: **Sergei, Sergeo.**

Serle: (Teutonic) "bearing arms; weapons."

Seth: (Hebrew) "chosen." Biblical: the son of Adam and Eve. The ancient Egyptian god of the sky, lord of the desert and warfare.

Seton: (Anglo-Saxon) "from the place by the sea."

Severino: (Latin) "firm on justice." Seve Ballesteros, golfer.

Severn: (Old English) "boundary." Severn Darden, actor.

Seward: (Anglo-Saxon) "defender of the coast."

Sewell: (Teutonic) "victorious on the sea."
Also: **Sewel.**

Sexton: (Middle English) "church official."

Seymour: (French) "follower of St. Maur." *See also* Maurice.

Shadow, Shadoe: a contem-porary name. Shadoe Stevens, television actor.

Shadwell: (Old English) "from the shed spring."
Also: **Shad.**

Shafir: (Aramaic-Hebrew) "fine; excellent; handsome."
Also: **Shifron.**

Shaheed: (Arabic) "witness, martyr."

Shalman: (Hebrew) "to be complete; to be rewarded."

Shamir: (Hebrew) "flint stone"; an Israeli place name.

Shamus: an Irish form of James.

Shanahan: (Irish Gaelic) "wise one."

Shandy: (Old English) "little boisterous one."

Shane: *see* John. Shane, romantic loner of 1949 novel and 1953 film of the same name; Shane Reynolds, baseball player.

Shanley: (Irish Gaelic) "old hero."

Shannon: (Irish Gaelic) "little old wise one." The longest river in Ireland.

Shattuck: (Middle English) "little shad fish."

Shaun: *see* Shawn. Shaun van Allen, hockey player.

Shaw: (Anglo-Saxon) "from the grove."

Shawn: an Irish form of John.

Shea: (Irish Gaelic) "majestic, scientific, ingenious one."

Shea Seals, basketball player.

Sheehan: (Irish Gaelic) "little peaceful one."

Sheffield: (Old English) "from the crooked field."

Shelby: *see* Selby. Shelby Foote, writer.

Sheldon: (Anglo-Saxon) "from the hill ledge; shelly valley." Sheldon Glashow, Nobel prize–winning physicist.
Also: **Shel, Shell, Shelly, Shelton.**

Shelley: (Anglo-Saxon) "from the ledge; shelly meadow."
Also: **Shel, Shell, Shelly.**

Shelton: (Old English) "from the ledge town." *See also* Sheldon.

Shem: (Hebrew) "renown."

Shen: (Chinese) "gentleman." Traditionally combined with another name.

Shepard: (Anglo-Saxon) "sheep tender."
Also: **Shep, Shepherd, Shepp, Sheppard.**

Shepley: (Anglo-Saxon) "of the sheep meadow."
Also: **Shep, Sheply.**

Sherard: (Anglo-Saxon) "a brave soldier."
Also: **Sherrard.**

Sherborne: (Old English) "from the clear brook."
Also: **Sherborn.**

Sheridan: (Celtic) "wild man; savage."
Also: **Sherry.**

Sherlock: (Old English) "a short-haired son."
Also: **Sherlocke.**

Sherman: (Anglo-Saxon) "wool shearer; sheep cutter."
Also: **Sherm.**

Sherrill: (Old English) "clear spring." Sherrill Milnes, opera singer.

Sherwin: (Anglo-Saxon) "a true friend." Sherwin Campbell Badger, ice skater (1901–1972).
Also: **Win, Wyn.**

Sherwood: (Anglo-Saxon) "bright forest." Sherwood Anderson, writer.
Also: **Wood, Woody.**

Shiloh: (Hebrew) "peace, abundance." City located near Jerusalem.

Shimon: (Hebrew) "to hear or be heard." Biblical: the second son of Jacob. Shimon Peres, Israeli foreign minister.

Shipley: (Old English) "dweller at the sheep meadow."

Shipton: (Old English) "dweller at the sheep estate."

Siddell: (Old English) "from the wide valley."

Sidney: (French) "a follower of Saint Denis." Sidney Lumet, film director.
Also: **Sid, Sidonio (Sp), Sydney.**

Sierra: (Latin) "saw-toothed mountain."

Sigfrid: (Teutonic) "glorious

peace." A hero of German myth.
Also: **Siegfried.**

Sigmund: (Teutonic) "victorious protector." Sigmund Freud, psychologist.

Sigurd: (Teutonic) "ruling spirit." Mythology: Sigurd the Volsung, Norse counterpart of the hero Siegfried.

Sigwald: (Old German) "victorious ruler."

Silas: (Latin) "of the forest"; abbreviation of Silvanus, the god of the woods. Silas Marner, hero of the George Eliot novel (1861).
Also: **Si, Silvan, Silvanus, Silvester, Sylvan, Sylvester.**

Silvano: (Latin) "of the forest."
Also: **Silvain, Silvanus.** See also Silas.

Simon: (Hebrew) "to be heard." Biblical: Simon Peter.
Also: **Si, Simeon.**

Simpson, Simson: see Samson.

Sinclair: (Latin) "saintly; shining light." Sinclair Lewis, Nobel prize–winning author.
Also: **Clair.**

Sing: (Hindi) "lion."

Sion: (Hebrew) "exalted."

Siward: (Teutonic) "conquering guardian."

Skelly: (Irish Gaelic) "storyteller."

Skelton: (Old English) "from the town on the ledge."

Skerry: (Old Norse) "from the rocky island."

Skipp: (Old Norse) "ship owner."
Also: **Skipper.**

Sky: a name from nature; Sky Masterson, character in a Damon Runyon story. See also Schuyler.

Slade: (Old English) "dweller in the valley."

Slevin: (Irish Gaelic) "mountaineer."
Also: **Slavin.**

Sloan: (Celtic) "warrior."
Also: **Sloane.**

Smedley: (Old English) "from the flat meadow."

Smith: (Old English) "blacksmith."

Snowden: (Old English) "from the snowy hill."

Snyder: (Teutonic) "tailor."

Sol: (Latin) "sun." The Roman god of the sun; a diminutive of Solomon. Sol Lewitt, artist.

Solomon: (Hebrew) "peaceable; wise." Solomon Burke, soul singer. Biblical: son of King David, and his successor.
Also: **Salomon, Sol, Solly.**

Solon: (Greek) "wise man."

Somerset: (Old English) "from the place of the summer settlers."

Somerton: (Old English) "from the summer estate."

Somerville: (Old Franco-German) "from the summer estate."

Sorrell: (Old French) "reddish-brown hair."

Southwell: (Old English) "from the south spring."

Spalding: (Old English) "from the split meadow." Spalding Gray, monologuist.

Spangler: (South German) "tinsmith."

Spark: (Middle English) "gay, gallant one." Spark Matsunaga, U.S. congressman.
Also: **Sparky.**

Spear: (Old English) "spearman."

Speed: (Old English) "success, prosperity."

Spencer: (French) "storekeeper; dispenser of provisions." Spencer Tracy, actor.
Also: **Spence, Spenser.**

Sprague: (Old English) "the quick one."
Also: **Sprage.**

Squire: (Middle English) "knight's attendant."

Stacy: (Latin) "stable companion." Stacy Keach, actor.
Also: **Stacey.**

Stafford: (Old English) "of the landing place."
Also: **Staffard, Staford.**

Stan: short form of Stanley and other names beginning Stan-.

Stanbury: (Old English) "from the stone fortress."

Stancliff: (Old English) "from the rocky cliff."

Standish: (Old English) "from the rocky park."

Stanfield: (Old English) "from the rocky field."

Stanford: (Anglo-Saxon) "of the stony crossing." Stanford White, architect.

Stanhope: (Old English) "from the stony vale."

Stanislaus: (Slavic) "glorious position." St. Stanislaus, patron saint of Poland. Stanislaus Zbyszko, wrestler.
Also: **Stanislav.**

Stanley: (Slavonic) "pride of the camp." Stanley Kubrick, filmmaker.
Also: **Lee, Stan, Stanleigh.**

Stanmore: (Old English) "from the rocky lake."

Stanton: (Anglo-Saxon) "from the stony place." Stanton Avery, American businessman.

Stanway: (Old English) "dweller on the paved stone road."

Stanwick: (Old English) "dweller at the rocky village."

Stanwood: (Old English) "dweller at the rocky forest."

Starling: (Old English) "starling bird."

Starr: (Middle English) "star."

Stedman: (Old English) "farmstead owner."
Also: **Steadman.**

Stefan: *see* Stephen. Stefan Edberg, tennis player.

Stein: (German) "stone."

Stephen: (Greek) "crown; garland." St. Stephen was the first king of Hungary.
Also: **Esteban, Estevan (Sp), Étienne (Fr), Stefan (Ger, Pol), Steffen, Stevan, Steve, Steven, Stevie, Václav (Slavic).**

Sterling: (Teutonic) "good value; honest; genuine." Sterling Brown, poet.
Also: **Stirling.**

Sterne: (Middle English) "austere one."
Also: **Stern.**

Steven: *see* Stephen.

Stewart: (Anglo-Saxon) "keeper of the estate."
Also: **Stew, Steward, Stu, Stuart.**

Stillman: (Anglo-Saxon) "quiet; gentle."

Stinson: (Old English) "son of stone."

Stockley: (Old English) "from the cleared meadow."

Stockton: (Old English) "from the farm in the clearing."

Stockwell: (Old English) "from the spring in the clearing."

Stoddard: (Anglo-Saxon) "keeper of horses."

Stoke: (Middle English) "village."

Stone: the English word used as a first name. Stone Phillips, broadcast journalist.
Also: **Stoney.**

Storm: (Old English) "tempest." Storm Field, weatherman.

Storr: (Old Norse) "great one."

Stowe: (Old English) "from the place."

Strahan: (Irish Gaelic) "wise man."

Stratford: (Old English) "river ford on the street."

Strong: (Old English) "powerful one."

Stroud: (Old English) "from the thicket."

Struthers, Strother: (Irish Gaelic) "from the stream." Strother Martin, actor.

Stuart: *see* Stewart.

Styles: (Old English) "dweller by the stiles."
Also: **Stiles.**

Suffield: (Old English) "from the south field."

Sullivan: (Irish Gaelic) "black-eyed one."

Sumner: (Latin) "the summoner." Sumner Redstone, executive.

Sutcliff: (Old English) "from the south cliff."
Also: **Southcliffe.**

Sutherland: (Old Norse) "from the southern land."

Sutton: (Anglo-Saxon) "from the south town; village."

Sven: (Scandinavian) "youth." Sven Nykvist, cinematographer.

Swaine: (Teutonic) "boy."
Also: **Swain, Swane.**

Sweeney: (Irish Gaelic) "little hero."

Swinton: (Old English) "dweller at the swine farm."

Sydney: *see* Sidney.

Sylvester: *see* Silas.

Symington: (Old English) "dweller at Simon's estate."

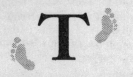

Tab: (Old German) "brilliant among the people."

Tad, Thad: *see* Theodore, Thaddeus.

Tadashi: (tah-DAH-shee) (Japanese) "loyal, faithful." Also: **Tad.**

Tadeo: (Aramaic) "praise."

Taffy: (Old Welsh) "beloved one."

Taggart: (Irish Gaelic) "son of the prelate."

Tai: (Chinese) "peaceful; in good health." Traditionally combined with a second name.

Tal: (Hebrew) "dew."

Talbott: (Anglo-Saxon) "bloodhound." Also: **Talbot, Tallboy.**

Taliesin: (Welsh) "radiant brow." The name of a 6th-century Welsh bard.

Tam, Tammany, Tomas: *see* Thomas.

Tama: (North American Indian) "a thunderbolt."

Tan: (Vietnamese) "new."

Tangier: the port city of northern Morocco. Tangier Smith, adventurer.

Tanka: (American Indian) "great."

Tanner: (Old English) "leather maker."

Tanton: (Old English) "from the quiet river town."

Tarik: (Arabic) "visitor." Also: **Taariq.**

Tarleton: (Old English) "thunder ruler's estate."

Tarquin: the name of two legendary kings of 6th-century Rome.

Tarrant: (Old Welsh) "thunder."

Tatanka: (Sioux Indian) "black buffalo."

Tate: (Teutonic) "cheerful." Tate Donovan, actor. Also: **Tait, Taite.**

Tavis: (Celtic) "son of David."

Taylor: (Latin) "the tailor." Tay Garnett, film director; Taylor Hackford, film director.

Teague: (Irish Gaelic) "poet."

Tearle: (Old English) "stern one."

Tecumseh: (American Indian) "who passes across space from one point to another; meteor; shooting star." Tecumseh, Indian chief; William Tecumseh Sherman, Union general.

Ted, Teddy: *see* Edward, Theodore, Theodoric.

Tedmond: (Old English) "national protector."
Also: **Tedman, Tedmund.**

Tedric: (Teutonic) "people's ruler."

Telford: (Old French) "iron-hewer."

Templeton: (Old English) "temple town."

Tennessee: an American Indian place name. Tennessee Williams, playwright.

Tennyson: (Middle English) "son of Dennis."
Also: **Tennison.**

Terence: (Latin) "tender."
Also: **Terrence, Terry, Torin, Torrance.**

Terrill: (Teutonic) "belonging to Thor." *See also* Tyrell.

Terris: (Old English) "son of Terrell or Terence."

Terry: *see* Terence. Terry Southern, screenwriter.

Thacher: *see* Thatcher.

Thaddeus: (Hebrew) "praise to God." Biblical: one of the 12 Apostles.
Also: **Tad, Tadeo (Sp), Thad.**

Thane: (Old English) "warrior attendant."

Thatcher, Thacher: (Anglo-Saxon) "a mender of roofs." Thacher Hurd, author, illustrator.
Also: **Thackeray, Thaxter.**

Thaw: (Old English) "ice thaw."

Thayer: (Teutonic) "of the nation's army."

Theo: short form of Theodore; also an independent name.

Theo Mizuhara, hip-hop disc jockey; Theo van Doesburg, Dutch painter.

Theobald: *see* Tybalt.

Theodore: (Greek) "gift of God."
Also: **Dore, Federico, Fedor, Feodor, Feodore, Tad, Ted, Teddie, Teddy, Teodor (Pol), Teodoro (Sp), Theo, Tudor.**

Theodoric: (Teutonic) "the people's ruler." Theodoric the Great, king of the Ostrogoths.
Also: **Derek, Derk, Derrick, Ted, Teddie, Teddy, Tedric.**

Theon: (Greek) "godly."

Theron: (Greek) "a hunter."

Thierry: (French) "people's ruler." Thierry Mugler, fashion designer.

Thomas: (Aramaic) "the twin." Biblical: one of the 12 disciples of Jesus. St. Thomas Aquinas.
Also: **Tammany, Thom, Thomasin, Tom, Tomas (Sp), Tomaso (It), Tomasz (Pol), Tommy.**

Thompson, Thomson: variants of Thomas.
Also: **Thomsen.**

Thor: (Scandinavian) "the thunderous one." Thor, god of war in Norse mythology. Thor Heyerdahl, adventurer.

Thorald: (Old Norse) "thunder ruler."
Also: **Thorold, Thorwald.**

Thorbert: (Old Norse) "thunder glorious."

Thorburn: (Old Norse) "thunder bear."

Thoreau: (Old French) "thunder water"; Henry David Thoreau, naturalist and writer.

Thorley: (Old English) "Thor's meadow."

Thormond: (Old English) "Thor's protection."

Thorndyke: (Old English) "from the thorny dike."

Thorne: (Old English) "dweller by a thorn tree."

Thornley: (Old English) "from the thorny meadow."

Thornton: (Anglo-Saxon) "from the thorny place." Thornton Wilder, playwright.

Thorpe: (Anglo-Saxon) "from the small village." Jim Thorpe, athlete.

Thulane: (origin uncertain) Thulane Malinga, boxer.

Thurgood: from the Norman surname. Thurgood Marshall, Supreme Court justice.

Thurlow: (Old English) "of Thor's mountain."
Also: **Thorlow.**

Thurman: (Scandinavian) "under Thor's protection." Thurman Thomas, football player.
Also: **Thorman.**

Thurston: (Scandinavian) "Thor's jewel; stone."
Also: **Thurstan.**

Tian: (Chinese) "to increase; tranquil." Traditionally combined with a second name.

Tiernan: (Irish Gaelic) "master."

Tierney: (Irish Gaelic) "lordly one." Tierney Malone, artist.

Tilden: (Anglo-Saxon) "from a fertile valley."

Tilford: (Old English) "from the good man's farm."

Tilton: (Old English) "from the liberal one's estate."

Tim: short form of Timothy.

Timon: (Greek) "reward, value."

Timothy: (Greek) "honoring God." Biblical: companion of Paul.
Also: **Tim, Timmie, Timmy.**

Tito: see Titus. Tito Puente, bandleader.

Titus: (Latin) "safe; saved."
Also: **Tito.**

Tobias: (Hebrew) "God's goodness." Tobias Wolff, writer.
Also: **Tobe, Tobit, Tobey, Toby.**

Todd: (Latin) "the fox."

Toft: (Old English) "a small farm."

Toland: (Old English) "owner of taxed land."

Tom, Tomas, Tommy: see Thomas.

Tomkin: (Old English) "little Tom."

Tony: see Anthony.

Toole: (Celtic) "lordly."
Also: **O'Toole.**

Tormey: (Irish Gaelic) "thunder spirit."

Torquil: (Scandinavian) "Thor's cauldron."

Torr: (Old English) "from the tower."

Torrance, Torin: *see* Terence. Also a Scottish place name.

Torrey: (Anglo-Saxon) "lofty eminence"; a Scottish place name.
Also: **Torry.**

Townley: (Old English) "from the town meadow."

Townsend: (Anglo-Saxon) "from the end of town."

Tracey: (Anglo-Saxon) "the brave defender."
Also: **Tracy.**

Trahern: (Old Welsh) "super strength."

Trainor: (Celtic) "champion."

Tranel: (origin uncertain) Tranel Hawkins, American track and field athlete.

Travis: (Latin) "from the crossroad." Travis Tritt, country singer.
Also: **Travers.**

Traylor: (Teutonic) "one who follows a clue."

Tredway: (Old English) "mighty warrior."

Tremayne: (Old Cornish) "dweller in the house at the rock."

Trent: (Latin) "swift."

Trevelyan: (Old Cornish) "from Elian's homestead."

Trevor: (Celtic) "careful traveler."
Also: **Trev.**

Trigg: (Old Norse) "trusty one."

Trinidad: (Latin) "triad, the Holy Trinity." Trini Lopez, singer/actor.

Tristan: (Latin) "sorrowful." Tristan and Isolde, the famous lovers of Celtic legend and inspirations for the opera by Wagner.
Also: **Trystan.**

Tristram: (Latin-Welsh) "sorrowful labor." Tris Speaker, baseball player.

Trowbridge: (Old English) "dweller by the tree bridge."

Troy: (Old French) "at the place of the curly-haired people." Troy Aikman, quarterback.

Truan: *see* True. Truan Monro, actor.

True: (Old English) "faithful, loyal one."

Truesdale: (Old English) "from the beloved one's farmstead."

Truman: (Anglo-Saxon) "a faithful man." Truman Capote, author.

Tucker: (Middle English) "a tucker of cloth."

Tudor: (Old Welsh) Welsh variation of Theodore.

Tully: (Irish Gaelic) "quiet, peaceful one."
Also: **Tulley.**

Tupper: (Old English) "sheep raiser."

Turner: (Latin) "worker with the lathe."

Turpin: (Old Norse) "thunder-Finn."

Tuxford: (Old Norse-English) "ford of the national spear-man."

Twain: (Middle English) "cut in two"; Mark Twain, author, humorist.

Twitchell: (Old English) "dweller on a narrow passage."

Twyford: (Old English) "from the double river ford."

Ty: A diminutive for any name beginning with Ty-. Also used as an independent name. Ty (Tyrus) Cobb, baseball player. *See also* Tye.

Tybalt: (Teutonic) "leader of the people." The character murdered by Romeo in Shakespeare's *Romeo and Juliet.*
Also: **Theobald, Thibaut, Ty, Tybald.**

Tye: (English) "dweller near the enclosure."

Tyler: (Anglo-Saxon) "maker of tiles or bricks."

Tynan: (Irish Gaelic) "dark or gray."

Tyrell: (Old English) "thunder ruler." Tyrell Biggs, boxer.
Also: **Terrell, Terrill.**

Tyrone: (Celtic) the name of an Irish county meaning "Owen's land." Tyrone Power, actor.
Also: **Ty.**

Tyson: (Teutonic) "son of the German." Tyson Wheeler, basketball player.
Also: **Sonny, Ty.**

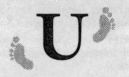

U

Udell: (Old English) "from the yew-tree valley."

Udolf: (Old English) "prosperous wolf."

Ugo: Italian form of Hugh.

Ulfred: (Old English) "peace of the wolf."

Ulger: (Old English) "wolf spear."

Ulmer: (Old Norse) "famous wolf."

Ulric, Ulrich: (Old German) "wolf-ruler." Ulrike Ottinger, film director.

Ulysses: (Greek) "angry one; wrathful." Ulysses S. Grant, general and 18th U.S. President.

Umar: (Arabic) "longevity."

Unger: (German) "from Hungary."
Also: **Ungar.**

Unni: (Hebrew) "modest."

Upton: (Anglo-Saxon) "from the hill town." Upton Sinclair, author.

Upwood: (Old English) "from the upper forest."

Urban: (Latin) "from the city; urbane, sophisticated."
Also: **Urbain, Urbano (It, Sp).**

Uriah: (Hebrew) "the Lord is my light." Biblical: the name of five different Old Testament characters.
Also: **Urias, Uriel.**

Usher: (English) "door-keeper."

Uziel: (Hebrew) "a mighty force."
Also: **Uzziel.**

Uzziah: (Hebrew) "God is strong."

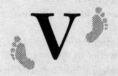

Vachel: (French) "keeper of the cattle." Vachel Lindsay, poet.
Also: **Vachil.**

Václav: *see* Stephen.

Vail: (Anglo-Saxon) "from the valley." Vail Johnson, jazz artist.
Also: **Vale, Valle.**

Val: (Teutonic) "might; power"; a short form of names beginning Val-. Val Kilmer, actor.

Valdemar: (Old German) "famous ruler."
Also: **Valdemere.**

Valentine: (Latin) "healthy; strong; valorous."
Also: **Val, Valente, Valentin, Valentino (It), Valentyn, Valiant.**

Valery, Valerian: (Latin) "strong; belonging to Valentine." Valéry Giscard d'Estaing, former president of France.

Valmont: (Teutonic) "protective power."

Van: (Dutch) "from Vander." Van Cliburn, pianist.

Vance: (Dutch) "the son of a famous family." Vance Brand, U.S. astronaut.
Also: **Van.**

Vanek: (Slavic) a form of Ivan.

Varian: (Latin) "clever; capricious."

Varun: (Hindi) "lord of the waters."

Vassily: (Slavic) "unwavering protector."
Also: **Vasili, Vass.**

Vaughan: (Celtic) "the small." Vaughn LeRoy Beals, CEO, Harley-Davidson.
Also: **Vaughn, Von, Vonn.**

Vedder: (Dutch) "father."

Vere: (Latin) "true; faithful." Vere Gordon Childe, British anthropologist.

Verge: (Anglo-French) "owner of a quarter-acre."

Vernal: (Latin) "spring."
Also: **Vernay.**

Verne: short form of Vernal, Vernon.

Verney: (Celtic) "a grove of alders."

Vernon: (Latin) "growing, flourishing." Vernon Jordan, civil rights leader.
Also: **Vern, Verne.**

Verrill: (Old French) "true one."

Victor: (Latin) "the conqueror." Victor Hugo, French novelist.
Also: **Vic, Vick, Victoir, Vittorio, Wiktor (Pol).**

Vigor: (Latin) "vigor."

Vincent: (Latin) "the conqueror." St. Vincent de Paul; Vincent van Gogh, artist.
Also: **Vin, Vince.**

Vinson: (Anglo-Saxon) "son of Vincent."

Virgil: (Latin) "strong; flourishing." Virgil Thomson, composer.
Also: **Vergil, Virg, Virgie, Virgy.**

Vito: (Latin) "vital." Vida Blue, baseball pitcher.
Also: **Vidal, Vitas, Vitus.**

Vivien: (Latin) "lively."
Also: **Vivian.**

Vladimir: (Slavonic) "the ruler of all"; a Russian place name. Vladimir Horowitz, pianist.
Also: **Vlad, Vladamir, Waldemar, Wladimir.**

Vladislav: (Old Slavic) "glorious ruler."

Volney: (Teutonic) "most popular."
Also: **Volny.**

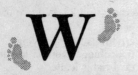

Waban: (American Indian) "the East Wind."

Wade: (Anglo-Saxon) "mover; wanderer." Wade Boggs, baseball player.

Wadley: (Old English) "the advancer's meadow."

Wadsworth: (Old English) "from Wade's castle."

Wagner: (German) "wagon maker."

Wainwright: (Old English) "wagon maker."

Waite: (Middle English) "guard." Waite Hoyt, baseball player.

Wake: (Old English) "watchful one."

Wakefield: (Old English) "dweller at the wet field."

Wakeley: (Old English) "from the wet field."

Wakeman: (Old English) "watchman."

Walbridge: (Teutonic) "dweller at the stone bridge."

Walby: (Old English) "from the walled dwellings."

Walcott: (Anglo-Saxon) "cottage dweller."

Waldemar: (Teutonic) "strong; famous."
Also: **Waldimar, Waldo.**

Walden: (Old English) "from the forest valley."

Waldo: (Old German) "ruler." Ralph Waldo Emerson, poet, essayist. *See also* Waldemar.

Waldron: (Old German) "ruling raven."

Walford: (Old English) "from the Welshman's ford."

Walfred: (Old German) "peaceful ruler."

Walker: (Anglo-Saxon) "forest walker." Walker Evans, photographer.

Wallace: (Teutonic) "the Welshman; stranger." Wallace Stegner, author.
Also: **Wallie, Wallis, Wally, Walsh.**

Waller: (Old English) "mason."

Wallis: see Wallace.

Walmond: (Old German) "ruling protector."

Walsh: see Wallace.

Walter: (Teutonic) "powerful; mighty warrior." Walter Cronkite, journalist.
Also: **Wallie, Wally, Walt, Walters.**

Walton: (Old English) "dweller at the town by a ruined Roman wall." Walton H. Walker, U.S. Army officer.

Walworth: (Old English) "from the Welshman's (stranger's) farm."

Walwyn: (Old English) "Welsh friend; friendly stranger."

Warburton: (Old English) "from the castle town."

Ward: (Anglo-Saxon) "watchman, guardian." Ward Goodenough, anthropologist.
Also: **Word.**

Wardell: (Old English) "from the watch hill."

Wardley: (Old English) "from the guardian's meadow."

Ware: (Anglo-Saxon) "always careful."

Warfield: (Middle English) "dweller at the field of the small stream dam."

Warford: (Middle English) "from the ford of the small stream dam."

Waring: (Anglo-Saxon) "the cautious soul."

Warley: (Middle English) "from the meadow of the small stream dam."

Warner: (Teutonic) "protecting warrior." Warner Baxter, actor.
Also: **Verner, Werner.**

Warren: (Teutonic) "game warden." Warren Beatty, actor, director.

Warrick: (Teutonic) "strong ruler."
Also: **Aurick, Vareck, Varick.**

Washburn: (Old English) "dweller at the flooding brook."

Washington: (Old English) "from the estate of the keen one's family." Washington Irving, author.

Watford: (Old English) "from the hurdle ford."

Watkins: (Old English) "son of Walter."

Watson: (Anglo-Saxon) "warrior's son."

Waverly: (Old English) "quaking aspen-tree meadow."

Wayland: (Teutonic) "from the land near the highway." Waylon Jennings, country singer.
Also: **Way, Waylan.**

Wayne: (Teutonic) "wagon

maker." Wayne Wang, film director.
Also: **Wain, Waine.**

Webster: (Anglo-Saxon) "weaver." Webb Pierce, country singer.
Also: **Web, Webb.**

Weddell: (Old English) "dweller at the advancer's hill."

Wei: (Chinese) "powerful; daring." Traditionally combined with a second name.

Welborne: (Old English) "dweller at the spring brook."

Welby: (Scandinavian) "from the farm by the spring."

Weldon: (Teutonic) "from a hill near the well."

Welford: (Old English) "from the spring ford."

Wellington: (Anglo-Saxon) "prosperous estate." The capital city of New Zealand.

Wells: (Old English) "from the spring."

Welton: (Old English) "dweller at the spring town."

Wenceslaus: (Old Slavic) "wreath of glory."

Wendell: (Teutonic) "wanderer." Oliver Wendell Holmes, Jr., Supreme Court justice.
Also: **Wendel.**

Wentworth: (Old English) "white one's estate."

Werner: (Old German) "de-fending army." Werner Herzog, filmmaker.
Also: **Verner, Warner.**

Wescott: (Teutonic) "dwells at west cottage."
Also: **Wes.**

Wesley: (Anglo-Saxon) "from the west meadow." Wesley Snipes, actor.
Also: **Wellesley, Wes, Westley.**

Wessel: (Teutonic) "from Wesel [Germany]." Wessell Anderson, jazz artist.

West: (Old English) "man from the West."

Westbrook: (Old English) "from the west brook."

Westby: (Old English) "from the west farmstead."

Weston: (Old English) "from the west estate." Weston Adams, hockey executive.

Wetherby: (Old English) "dweller at the wether [sheep] farm."

Wetherell: (Old English) "from the corner where white sheep grazed in green pastures."

Wetherly: (Old English) "dweller at the sheep meadow."

Wharton: (Old English) "estate at the embankment."

Wheatley: (Old English) "wheat field."

Wheaton: (Old English) "wheat town."

Wheeler: (Old English) "wheel maker."

Whistler: (Old English) "piper."

Whit: short form of names beginning Whit-. Whit Stillman, filmmaker.

Whitby: (Old English) "from the white farmstead."

Whitcomb: (Old English) "from the white hollow."

Whitelaw: (Anglo-Saxon) "of the white hill."

Whitfield: (Old English) "from the white field."

Whitford: (Old English) "from the white ford."

Whitlock: (Old English) "man with a white lock of hair."

Whitman: (Old English) "white-haired man"; Walt Whitman, poet.

Whitmore: (Old English) "from the white moor."

Whitney: (Anglo-Saxon) "from a white island."

Whittaker: (Old English) "dweller at the white field."

Wickham: (Old English) "from the village meadow."

Wickley: (Old English) "village meadow."

Wilbert, Wilbur: see Gilbert. Wilbur Shaw, race car driver.

Wiley: (Anglo-Saxon) "beguiling." Wiley Post, aviator. Also: **Wylie.**

Wilford: (Old English) "ford near the willows." Wilford Brimley, actor.

Wilfred: (Teutonic) "firm peacemaker." St. Wilfrid. Also: **Fred, Freddie.**

Wilkins: a form of William.

Wilkins Micawber, kindhearted gentleman in Dickens' *David Copperfield.*

Will, Willy: *see* William.

Willard: (Old English) "resolute and brave." Willard van Dyke, photographer, filmmaker (1906–1986).

Willem: Dutch form of William. Willem de Kooning, artist.

William: (Teutonic) "determined protector." William the Conqueror, king of England.
Also: **Bill, Billie, Billy, Guillaume (Fr), Guillermo (Sp), Wilhelm, Will, Willet, Willis, Willy, Wilson.**

Willis: a form of William, Wilson.

Willoughby: (Old English) "from the willow farm."

Wills: a form of William.

Wilmer: (Old German) "famous, resolute one."

Wilmot: (Old German) "resolute spirit."

Wilson: (Teutonic) "son of William." Wilson Pickett, soul singer.
Also: **Wil.**

Wilton: (Old English) "from the spring farm." Wilt Chamberlain, basketball player.

Win: short form of names beginning Win-. *See also* Wynn.

Winchell: (Old English) "from a bend in a piece of land."

Windsor: (Old English) "boundary bank."

Winfield: (Anglo-Saxon) "from the friendly field." Winfield Scott, U.S. Army general.

Wingate: (Old English) "divine protection."

Winifred: (Teutonic) "friend of peace."
Also: **Fred, Win, Winfred, Winfrid.**

Winslow: (Teutonic) "from the friendly hill." Winslow Homer, painter.
Also: **Win.**

Winston: (Anglo-Saxon) "from the friendly town." Winston Churchill, British prime minister.
Also: **Win, Winton.**

Winter: (Old English) "born in winter."

Winthrop: (Teutonic) "from the friendly village."

Winton: (Old English) "from the friend's estate." Wynton Marsalis, jazz trumpet player.
Also: **Witton.**

Winward: (Old English) "friend's forest."

Wirt: (German) "master."

Witt: see Witter.

Witter: (Old English) "wise warrior."

Witton: (Old English) "from the wise man's estate."

Woden: (Teutonic) "furious warrior."

Wolcott: (Old English) "from the wolf's cottage."

Wolfe: (Teutonic) "a wolf." Wolf Larsen, ship's captain in Jack London novel *The Sea Wolf* (1904).
Also: **Wulff.**

Wolfgang: (Old German) "advancing wolf." Wolfgang Amadeus Mozart, composer.

Wolfram: (Teutonic) "respected; feared."

Wladimir: see Vladimir.

Woodley: (Anglo-Saxon) "from the wooded meadow."

Woodman: (Anglo-Saxon) "woodcutter."

Woodrow: (Anglo-Saxon) "from the hedgerow in the wood." Woody Guthrie, singer/songwriter (1912–1967).
Also: **Woodie.**

Woodruff: (Old English) "forest warden."

Woodson: (Old English) "Wood's son."

Woodward: (Old English) "forester."

Woody: short form of names beginning Wood-. Woody Allen, filmmaker.

Worcester: (Old English) "alder-forest army camp."

Word: see Ward.

Wordsworth: (Old English) "wolf guardian's farm."

Worth: (Old English) "farmstead."

Worton: (Old English) "dweller at the vegetable farm."

Wray: (Old Norse) "from the corner property."

Wren: (Old Welsh) "chief." Also: **Wrenn.**

Wright: (Anglo-Saxon) "craftsman; worker." Wright Morris, writer, photographer.

Wyatt: (Teutonic) "lively." Wyatt Earp, Western hero (1848–1929). *See also* Guy.

Wyborn: (Old Norse) "war bear."

Wycliff: (Old English) "from the white cliff."

Wylie: (Anglo-Saxon) "beguiling; charming." Also: **Wiley.**

Wyman: (Old English) "warrior."

Wymer: (Old English) "famous in battle."

Wyndham: (Old English) "from the enclosure with the winding path."

Wynn: (Old Welsh) "white one." Wynn Bullock, photographer. Also: **Wynne.** *See also* Elwin.

Wynton: *see* Winton.

Wythe: (Middle English) "dweller at the willow tree."

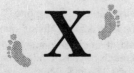

Xander: a form of Alexander. Xander Berkeley, actor.

Xavier: (Arabic) "bright." Xavier Cugat, bandleader. Also: **Javier, Zavier.**

Xenos: (Greek) "stranger."

Xerxes: (Persian) "king." Xerxes I, king of Persia.

Xian: (Chinese) "virtuous; celebrated." Traditionally combined with a second name.

Xylon: (Greek) "from the forest."

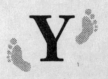

Yale: (Teutonic) "payer; yielder." Yale Lary, football player.

Yan: (Chinese) "ablaze." Traditionally combined with a second name.

Yancy: (French) "Englishman." Also: **Yancey.**

Yang: (Chinese) "the sun." Traditionally combined with a second name.

Yardley: (Teutonic) "dweller at the meadow pasture."

Yates, Yeats: (Anglo-Saxon) "the gate dweller; protector." The name honors the Irish poet William Butler Yeats.

Yehudi: (Hebrew) "the praise of the Lord." Yehudi Menuhin, violinist.

Yeoman: (Middle English) "retainer."

Yin: (Chinese) "musical sound." Traditionally combined with a second name.

York: (Latin) "sacred tree"; a family name and British place name.
Also: **Yorick, Yorke.**

Yoshi: (YOH-shee) (Japanese) "fine, splendid."

Yul: (Mongolian) "beyond the horizon." Yul Brynner, actor.

Yule: (Old English) "born at Christmas."
Also: **Yules.**

Yuma: (American Indian) "son of a chief."

Yuri: Russian variant of George. Yuri Gagarin, Soviet cosmonaut.
Also: **Youri.**

Yusef: (Arabic) Joseph.

Yves: (Scandinavian) "an archer." Yves Saint Laurent, fashion designer.
Also: **Ives, Yvon.**

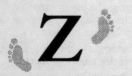

Zabdiel: (Hebrew) "God endows."

Zachariah: (Hebrew) "the Lord's remembrance." Zachariah Chandler, U.S. senator.
Also: **Zac, Zach, Zacharias, Zachary, Zack.**

Zachary: see Zachariah.

Zachary Taylor, 12th U.S. President.

Zack: see Zachariah.

Zadok: (Hebrew) "righteous one."

Zale: (Greek) "surge of the sea."

Zander: a form of Alexander. Zander Hollander, writer.
Also: **Zandor.**

Zane: see John. Zane Grey, Western writer.

Zared: (Hebrew) "ambush."

Zavier: see Xavier.

Zebadiah: (Hebrew) "the Lord's gift."
Also: **Zeb, Zebe, Zebedee.**

Zebulon: (Hebrew) "dwelling place." Zebulon Pike, explorer.
Also: **Lonny, Zeb.**

Zedekiah: (Hebrew) "justice of the Lord."

Zeeman: (Dutch) "seaman."

Zeke: see Ezekiel.

Zelig: (Teutonic) "blessed."
Also: **Selig.**

Zelotes: (Greek) "zealous one."

Zenas: (Greek) "Jupiter's gift."

Zephaniah: (Hebrew) "the Lord is my secret."
Also: **Zeph.**

Zeus: (Greek) "living one."

Ziv: (Old Slavic) "living one."

Zola: (French) surname of French novelist Emile Zola used as a first name.

Zuriel: (Hebrew) "God; my rock."

NAMES FOR GIRLS

NAMES FOR GIRLS

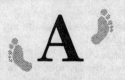

Abby: *see* Abigail.
Also: **Abbe, Abbey.**

Abey: (American Indian—Omaha) "leaf."

Abigail: (Hebrew) "my father rejoices." Biblical: the beautiful wife of King David.
Also: **Abbey, Abbie, Abby, Gael, Gail, Gale, Gayle.**

Abra: (Hebrew) feminine of Abraham.

Abrona: (Latin) a Roman goddess who presided over departures.

Acacia: (Greek) the tropical acacia tree symbolizes resurrection.
Also: **Casey.**

Acantha: (Greek) "sharp-pointed."

Ada: (Old English) "joyous." Ada Louise Huxtable, architecture critic; Ada, the computer language.
Also: **Addie, Addy, Aida.**

Adabella: "joyous and beautiful"; combination of Ada and Bella.
Also: **Adabelle.**

Adah: (Hebrew) "ornament."

Adalia: (Old German) "noble one."

Adamae: combination of Ada and Mae, q.v. Ada and May.

Adamina: (Latin) feminine of Adam.

Adar: (Hebrew) "fire"; the sixth month of the Jewish year.

Addie, Addy: short form of Adelaide and other names beginning Ad-.

Adela, Adele: *see* Adelaide.

Adelaide: (Latin/German) "noble and of kind spirit." Adelaide, the capital city of South Australia.
Also: **Adalia, Adaline, Addy, Adelaida (Sp), Adele, Adelia, Adelicia, Adelina, Adeline, Adella, Adila, Delia, Della.**

Adeline: a form of Adelaide. Adelina Pena, opera singer.
Also: **Adalina, Adaline, Adalyn, Addy.**

Adelphe: (Greek) "beloved sister."

Adi: (Hebrew) "adornment."
Also: **Adie.**

Adina: (Hebrew) "slender."
Also: **Adena, Adinah.**

Admire: one of the Puritan names.

Adonia: (Greek) "beautiful or godlike." Feminine of Adonis.

Adonica: (Latin) "sweet."
Also: **Adoncia.**

Adora: (Latin) "the beloved; the adored."
Also: **Adoree, Dora, Doria.**

Adorna: (Latin) "she beautifies."

Adria: *see* Adrienne.

Adriana: *see* Adrienne.

Adrienne: (Latin) "from Adria." Adrienne Rich, poet.
Also: **Adrena, Adria, Adrian, Adriana, Adriane, Adrianne.**

Aeron: (Welsh) "fruit; berry."
Also: **Aerona.**

Africa, Afrika: (Gaelic) "pleasant." The origin of the name of the continent Africa is unclear.

Agatha: (Greek) "good." Agatha Christie, mystery writer.
Also: **Agathe (Fr), Agethe, Aggie, Aggy.**

Agila: (Latin) "active of mind and body."

Agnes: (Greek) "pure, chaste." St. Agnes; Agnes de Mille, choreographer.
Also: **Aggie, Aggy, Agness, Nessa, Nessie, Ines, Inez (Sp).**

Agni: (Hindi) the fire goddess in Hindu mythology.

Ah lan: (Chinese) "orchid."

Aida: *see* Ada.

Aidan: (Irish Gaelic) "little fire."

Aileen: (Greek) "light."
Also: **Aleen, Alene, Aline, Eileen, Ileana, Ilene.**

Ailsa: (Teutonic) "girl of cheer."

Aimee: (French) "beloved." Aimee Semple McPherson, evangelist.

Airlia: (Greek) "of the air; ethereal."

Aisha: (Arabic) "life." Aisha was the favorite wife of the prophet Mohammed.
Also: **Aesha, Ayeisha.** *See also* Asia.

Akemi: (ah-KEH-mee) (Japanese) "bright; beautiful."

Aki: (AH-kee) (Japanese) "autumn." Akiko Yosana, Japanese poet.
Also: **Akiko.**

Alabretta: (Greek) "white pearl."

Alama: (Swahili) "a sign."

Alameda: (Spanish) "poplar tree."

Alana: (Celtic) "fair, handsome." Feminine of Alan. Alanis Morissette, rock singer.
Also: **Alannah, Alayne, Alina, Allana, Lana, Lane.**

Alani: (Hawaiian) a fragrant species of tree.

Alaudine: (Latin) "the lark."

Alberta: (Teutonic) "noble; bright." Feminine of Albert. Alberta Hunter, blues singer.
Also: **Albertine, Allie, Bert, Berta, Bertie, Elberta, Elbertine.**

Alcina: (Greek) "strong-minded."
Also: **Alcena.**

Alda: (Teutonic) "happy; rich."

Aldis: (Old English) "from the oldest house."
Also: **Alda, Aldas, Aldya, Aldys.**

Aldona: (Spanish) "wise."

Aldora: (Greek) "winged gift."

Alejandra: Spanish form of Alexandria. Feminine of Alejandro.

Alene: see Aileen.

Alesia: (Greek) "helper."

Alethea: (Greek) "truth." In mythology, the goddess of truth.
Also: **Aleta, Alithea, Alitta, Letta, Thea.**

Aletta: a form of Alethea. Dr. Aletta Jacobs, Holland's first woman physician (1854–1929).
Also: **Alette.**

Alexandra: (Greek) "helper of humankind." Feminine of Alexander.
Also: **Alejandra (Sp), Alessandra (It), Alex, Alexa, Alexandrine, Alexia, Alexis, Alix, Alla, Elexa, Sacha, Sandi, Sandra, Sascha, Sasha, Sondra.**

Alexis: see Alexandra.

Alfarata: a coined name from a 19th-century song.
Also: **Alphareta, Alpharetta.**

Alfonsine: (Teutonic) "noble and battle-ready."
Also: **Alfonsina.**

Alfreda: (German) "elf counselor."
Also: **Alfie, Elfrida, Frida.**

Ali: a form of Alice and other names beginning Al-. (Arabic) "greatest." Ali MacGraw, actress.

Alice: (Greek) "truth."
Also: **Ailsa (Scot), Alicia (It, Sp), Alisa, Alison, Alissa, Alla, Allie, Ally, Alyce, Alys, Alysia, Alyssa, Elissa, Elke.**

Alicia: Spanish form of Alice. Alicia Alonzo, ballerina.

Alida: (Greek) "beautifully dressed."
Also: **Aleda, Lita.**

Alima: (Arabic) "learned in dance and music."

Alina: see Adeline. Aline Bernstein, theatrical designer.

Alison: see Alice.

Allard: (Old English) "sacred and brave."

Allegra: (Latin) "cheerful." Allegra Kent, ballerina.
Also: **Alegria, Allegria.**

Allie, Ally: short forms of names beginning Al-.
Also: **Alley.**

Allyn: a form of Allen.

Alma: (Hebrew) "young woman." (Italian) "soul." (Latin) "loving, nurturing." Alma Gluck, opera singer.

Almah: (Arabic) "learned."

Almira: (Arabic) "princess."
Also: **Elmira.**

Aloha: (Hawaiian) "love; compassion; mercy; regards; to greet, bid farewell."

Alona: (Hebrew) "oak tree."
Also: **Allona.**

Aloysia: (Teutonic) "famed

battler." Feminine of Aloysius.
Also: **Aloise, Aloisia, Aloyse, Lois.**

Alpha: (Greek) "first one" the first letter of the Greek alphabet.
Also: **Alfa.**

Alsatia: (German) "from Alsace."

Alta: (Latin) "tall in spirit."

Altagracia: (Latin) "our lady of Altagracia."

Althea: (Greek) "wholesome, healing." Althea Gibson, tennis player.
Also: **Altheda, Althee, Altheta, Thea.**

Alura: (Old English) "divine counselor."

Alva: (Latin) "fair one."

Alverna: (French) "all green; flourishing."
Also: **Alverda.**

Alvina: (Teutonic) "beloved; friend of all." Feminine of Alvin.
Also: **Vina.**

Alvira: (Teutonic) "elfin arrow."

Alyssa: (Greek) "logical"; a flower name, alyssum. Alysiah Bond, basketball player.
Also: **Alissa, Alysa, Elissa.**

Alzena: (Arabic-Persian) "the woman."
Also: **Alzina.**

Ama: (Latin) "loved one."
Also: **Amabel, Amabella, Amabelle.**

Amabel: see Ama.

Amal: (Arabic) "hope." (Hebrew) "work."
Also: **Amala.**

Amalia: see Amelia.

Amanda: (Latin) "lovable."
Also: **Manda, Mandie, Mandy.**

Amani: (Swahili) "peace."

Amara: (Greek) "eternal beauty."

Amarantha: (Greek) a flower name.
Also: **Amaranth.**

Amaris: (Latin) "moon child."

Amaryllis: (Latin) a flower name.
Also: **Maryllis.**

Amaya: (Sanskrit) "guileless."

Amber: (Arabic) the semiprecious gemstone made up of petrified resin and said to have magical healing properties.
Also: **Amberly.**

Ambrosine: (Greek) "divine."
Also: **Ambrosina.**

Amei: (AH-may) (Chinese) "plum blossom; beautiful."

Amelia: (Teutonic) "industrious." Amelia Earhart, aviatrix; Amelita Galli-Curci, opera singer.
Also: **Amalia (Sp), Amelie (Fr), Ameline, Emblem, Emmeline, Melie, Mell, Mill, Millie.** See also Emily.

Amelinda: (Latin-Spanish) "beloved and pretty."

Amethyst: (Greek) the purple quartz crystal whose energy is said to restore calm.

Ami, Amie: variant spellings of Amy.

Amina: (Arabic/Swahili) "faithful." Mother of Mohammed; Nigerian queen.
Also: **Ameena.**

Aminita: (American Indian) "a fawn."
Also: **Amenita.**

Amity: (Old French) "friendship."
Also: **Amita (It).**

Amy: (Latin) "beloved." Amy Lowell, poet.
Also: **Aimee, Amie, Esme.**

An: (Chinese) "peace."

Ana: variant of Ann, Hanna.
Also: **Anabel, Anabella, Anabelle.**

Anais: (French/Greek) "fruitful." Anais Nin, French author.

Anastasia: (Greek) "resurrection."
Also: **Ana, Anastassia, Stacey, Stacy, Tasia.**

Anatola: (Greek) "of the East." Feminine of Anatole.

Andee: see Andrea. Andie MacDowell, actress.

Andrea: (Latin) "womanly." Feminine of Andrew.
Also: **Andee, Andi, Andra, Andreana, Andree, Andria, Andriana, Andy.**

Anemone: (Greek) "wind flower." According to Greek myth, anemones sprang from the passionate tears shed by Venus over the body of the slain Adonis. Also, a nymph named Anemone was transformed into a spring flower by the goddess Flora, enraged with jealousy because Anemone was loved by Zephyr, the gentle West Wind.

Angela: "angelic; heavenly messenger."
Also: **Angel, Angelika, Angeliki, Angelina, Angeline, Angelique, Angelita, Angie, Anjelica.**

Angelica: Anjelica Huston, actress. See also Angela.

Angie: see Angela.

Anica: a form of Ann.

Anika, Annika: forms of Ann.

Anisia: see Anysia.
Also: **Anissa.**

Anita: Spanish form of Ann. Anita Loos, screenwriter.

Anjanette: combination of Ann and Jeanette.

Ann: (Hebrew) "full of grace, mercy, and prayer." Originally from the name Hannah. St. Anne; Ann Richards, governor of Texas.
Also: **Ana, Anabel, Anabella, Anabelle, Anica, Anika, Anita (Sp), Anna, Anne, Annetta, Annette, Annie, Annika, Annora, Anya, Hannah, Hannie, Nan, Nana, Nancy, Nanete, Nanette (Fr), Nanine, Nanon, Nina, Ninette, Ninon.**

Anna: a form of Ann. Anna Pavlova, ballerina.

Annabelle: see Ann.

Annabeth: combination of Anna and Beth. Annabeth Gish, actress.

Annalise: a combination of Anna and Lisa.
Also: **Annalisa, Annelisa, Annelise.**

Annamaria: a combination of Anna and Maria.
Also: **Anna-maria, Annemarie.**

Annette: *see* Ann.

Annika: *see* Ann. Annika Sorenstam, golfer.

Annunciata: (Latin) "announced; a messenger."
Also: **Nunciata.**

Anouk: Russian form of Ann. Anouk Aimée, French actress.

Anselma: (Teutonic) "the protectress."
Also: **Selma, Zelma.**

Ansonia: feminine of Anson.

Anthea: (Greek) "like a flower."

Antoinette: *see* Antonia.

Antonia: (Latin) "priceless." Feminine of Anthony. Title character in the Willa Cather novel *My Antonia.*
Also: **Antoinetta, Antoinette (Fr), Antoni, Antonina, Netta, Nettie, Netty, Toinette, Toni, Tony.**

Anya: *see* Ann.

Anysia: (Greek) "complete."

Aphra: (Greek) "sea foam." Aphra Behn, British playwright.

Aphrodite: in Greek mythology, the beautiful goddess of love.

Apolline: (Greek) "sun or sunlight." Apollonia, singer.

April: (Latin) "to open"; the spring month.
Also: **Aprile, Aprilette, Aprili, Averell, Avril.**

Aquilina: (Spanish) "eagle." Feminine of Aquilino.

Arabella: (Latin) "fair and beautiful altar." Arabella Mansfield Bobb, first woman admitted to the bar (1869).
Also: **Arabela, Arabelle, Bella, Belle.**

Arcadia: (Spanish) "adventurous woman"; an idyllic region or pastoral setting, derived from the ancient Greek word representing a rural paradise in Greek and Roman poetry. Arcadia Baker, philanthropist.

Arcelia: (Spanish) "treasure chest."

Ardea: (Latin) "a heron."
Also: **Ardeen.**

Ardelle: *see* Ardis.

Arden: *see* Ardis.

Ardis: (Latin) "fervent, eager."
Also: **Ardelia, Ardelis, Ardella, Ardelle, Arden.**

Arela, Arella: (Hebrew) "angel; messenger."

Aretha: (Greek) "virtuous ruler"; a name popularized by Aretha Franklin, rhythm and blues singer.
Also: **Areta, Aretina.**

Argene: (French) "silvery."
Also: **Arjean.**

Aria: (Latin) "a solo melody."

Ariadne: (Greek) "holy one." Mythology: the daughter of King Midas.
Also: **Aria, Ariadna, Ariana, Ariane.**

Ariana: *see* Ariadne.

Ariel: (Hebrew) "lion of God"; the "airy" spirit of Shakespeare's *Tempest*. Ariel Durant, historian, writer.
Also: **Ariela, Ariella.**

Arizona: (American Indian) meaning unclear; possibly "little creeks" or "silver-bearing."

Arlene: (Celtic) "pledge." Arlene Croce, dance critic.
Also: **Arlana, Arleen, Arlena, Arlette, Arlina, Arline, Arlyn, Lena, Lina.**

Arlo: (Latin) "the barberry bush."

Arlys: (Teutonic) "a pledge."

Armida: (Latin) "little armed one."

Armina: (Old German) "warrior maid."
Also: **Armine, Ermine.**

Arnalda: (Old German) "strong as an eagle." Feminine form of Arnold.
Also: **Arnelle.**

Arnelle: feminine form of Arnold.

Artemisia: (Greek, Spanish) Mythology: the Greek goddess of the hunt and, in late mythology, the moon. Also a plant name. Artemisia Gentileschi, Italian painter (1593–1652).
Also: **Artemis.**

Asher: (Hebrew) "fortunate."

Ashley: (English) "meadow of ash trees." Ashley Judd, actress.
Also: **Ashely, Ashleigh, Ashly.**

Ashlin: (Old English) "dweller at the ash-tree pool."

Ashling: (Celtic) "dream; vision."

Asia: (contemporary) the name of the continent.

Asta: (Greek) "star." *See also* Aster, Astra.

Aster: (Greek) "star; a flower with a yellow center and multipetaled rays."
Also: **Asta.**

Astra: (Greek) "like a star." Astraea, Greek goddess of justice who disseminated virtue among mankind.
Also: **Astrea, Astred, Astrid.**

Astraea: *see* Astra.

Astrid: (Norse) "divine beauty."
Also: **Astred.**

Atalie: (Swiss) "pure."

Athena: (Greek) "wise; wisdom." Mythology: the Greek goddess of wisdom, fertility, and warfare.
Also: **Athene.**

Aubrey: (Teutonic) "elf ruler."
Also: **Aubree, Aubry.**

Audra: variant of Audrey.

Audrey: (English) "strong, noble." Audrey Hepburn, actress.
Also: **Audie, Audra, Audre, Audriana, Audrianna, Audrie, Audry, Dee.**

Augusta: (Latin) "exalted; majestic." Feminine of August.
Also: **Augustina, Augustine, Austin, Austina, Austine, Gussie, Gusta.**

Aurelia: (Latin) "golden."
Also: **Aura, Aurel, Aurelie, Auria, Aurie, Ora, Oralia, Oralie, Orelia.**

Aurora: (Latin) "dawn." Mythology: Roman goddess of the dawn.
Also: **Aurore, Rori, Rorie, Rory.**

Austin: a form of Augusta.
Also: **Austen.**

Autumn: (Latin) "autumn." Autumn Roxanne Burke, daughter of Yvonne Braithwaite Burke, congresswoman.

Ava: see Avis.

Avalon: the mysterious island of Arthurian legend.

Avelina: (Latin) "from Avellino."

Avis: "a bird."
Also: **Ava, Avi, Avice.**

Avril: French form of April. Avril Angers, British actress.

Ayeisha: see Aisha.

Ayla: (Hebrew) "oak tree." Ayla, heroine of the novel *The Clan of the Cave Bear*, by Jean M. Auel.

Ayn: see Ann. Ayn Rand, novelist.

Azalea: a flower name.

Azarine: (Teutonic) "noble woman."
Also: **Azarena, Azarina.**

Aziza: (Arabic) "precious."
Also: **Azize.**

Azura: (French) "sky-blue."
Also: **Azora, Azure.**

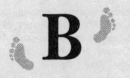

B

Babette: see Barbara.

Babe: short form of Barbara; also a nickname. Mildred (Babe) Didrikson, athlete.

Bambi: (Italian) "child." The baby deer of the Disney movie and 1926 novel of the same name.
Also: **Bambalina, Bambino.**

Bao: (Chinese) "bud." Traditionally combined with another name.

Barbara: (Greek) "the stranger." Barbara Bush, First Lady of the U.S.; Barbara McClintock, botanist.
Also: **Babe, Babette, Babs, Barbery, Barbette, Barbra, Barby, Bobbi, Bobbie.**

Basha: (Swahili) "act of God." (Polish) "the stranger." Basia, pop singer.

Basilia, Basilea: (Greek) "regal." The mythological Basilea was the daughter of Coelus and Terra, heaven and earth, and the mother of all the gods.
Also: **Basille (Fr).**

Bathsheba: (Hebrew) "the daughter of our oath." Biblical: Bathsheba was the beautiful wife of Uriah seduced by David.
Also: **Sheba.**

Batista: (Greek) "the baptized."
Also: **Baptista.**

Bea, Bee: short forms of Beatrice. Bea Arthur, actress.

Beata: (Latin) "blessed; divine."
Also: **Bea.**

Beatrice, Beatrix: (Latin) "she brings joy." Beatrice, queen of the Netherlands; Beatrix Potter, author, illustrator.
Also: **Bea, Beata, Beatriz (Sp), Bebe, Bee, Trixie.**

Beatriz: a Spanish form of Beatrice.

Bebe: a form of Beatrice; also an independent name. Bebe Moore Campbell, writer.

Becky: see Rebecca.

Bee: short form of Beatrice also used as an independent name.

Bela: (Hebrew) "God's oath." (Hungarian) "nobly bright." (Hindustani) "a fragrant jasmine."

Belinda: (Latin) "beautiful."
Also: **Bel, Linda, Lindy.**

Belisaria: (German) "the swordsman."

Bellanca: (Italian) "blond one."

Belle: (French) "beautiful." Belle Sherwin, suffragist; Belle Starr, outlaw.
Also: **Belita, Bella (It).** See also Arabella, Isabel, Mabel.

Bena: (Hebrew) "wise."

Benedicta: (Latin) "one who is blessed." Feminine of Benedict.
Also: **Benedetta, Benetta, Benicia, Benita.**

Benita: see Benedicta. Benita Valente, opera singer.

Berenice: see Bernice.

Bernadette: (French) "brave like a bear." Feminine of Bernard. St. Bernadette of Lourdes; Bernadette Peters, actress.
Also: **Bernadine, Bernadina (It, Sp), Bernetta, Bernie, Bernita.**

Bernice, Berenice: (Greek) "she brings victory." Berenice Abbott, photographer.
Also: **Bernette, Bernie, Berny.**

Berry: (English) "berry"; a French place name (Berri).

Bertha: (Teutonic) "shining; bright." Mythology: the Teutonic goddess of fertility. Berthe Morisot, French Impressionist painter; Bertha Suttner, first woman to win the Nobel Peace Prize.
Also: **Berta, Berthe (Fr), Bertie, Bertina, Birdie.**

Bertilde: (Old English) "shining battle maid."

Bertrade: (Old English) "shining counselor."

Beryl: (Greek) a mineral and prized gemstone of varying colors, from deep emerald green to aquamarine blue, golden yellow, and red. Beryl Markham, aviatrix and author of *West with the Night,* who was the first person to fly solo across the Atlantic from east to west.
Also: **Berrie, Berry, Beryle.**

Bess, Bessie: see Elizabeth. Bessie Smith, "Queen of the

Blues"; Bess Truman, First Lady of the U.S.

Beth: (Hebrew) "house of God."
Also: **Bethany, Bethel.** See also Elizabeth.

Bethany: a biblical place name.

Betsy, Betsey: a familiar form of Elizabeth. Betsey Johnson, fashion designer.

Bette: variant of Betty. Bette Davis, actress; Bette Midler, singer-actress.

Bettina: a form of Betty. Bettina von Arnim, German writer (1785–1859).

Betty: short form of Elizabeth.

Beulah: (Hebrew) "she who will be married." Biblical: a place name for Israel.

Beverly: (Anglo-Saxon) "dweller at the beaver meadow." Beverly Sills, opera singer, director of the New York City Opera.
Also: **Bev, Beverley.**

Bevin: (Irish Gaelic) "melodious lady."

Bian: (Vietnamese) "to be hidden."

Bianca: (Italian) "white." Bianca Jagger, former wife of the Rolling Stones' Mick Jagger.
Also: **Biancha.** See also Blanche.

Billie: (Old English) "determination." Billie Holiday, singer; Billie Jean King, tennis player.

Bin: (Chinese) "refined."

Bina: (Latin) "kind."

Birdie: (English) "sweet little bird."

Birgit, Birgitta: variants of Bridget.

Blaine: (Gaelic) "thin, lean."
Also: **Blane, Blayne.**

Blair: (Gaelic) "dweller on the plain." Blair Brown, actress.

Blake: (Old English) "dark; dark complexion."

Blanche: (French) "fair; white." Blanche DuBois, unforgettable character in A Streetcar Named Desire, by Tennessee Williams; Blanche Knopf, editor, publisher.
Also: **Bellanca, Bianca (It), Blanca (Sp).**

Blessing: (Old English) "consecrated one."

Bliss: (Old English) "gladness, joy." See also Blythe.

Blondina: (Old French) "fair one."
Also: **Blondine.**

Blossom: (Old English) "fresh, lovely." Blossom Dearie, cabaret singer. See also Flora.

Blythe: (Anglo-Saxon) "cheerful; happy." Blythe Danner, actress.
Also: **Blithe.**

Bo: (Chinese) "precious."

Bobbi, Bobbie: see Roberta.

Bonfilia: (Italian) "good daughter."

Bonita: (Spanish) "pretty."

Bonnie: (Middle English) "good." Bonnie Blair, first

American woman to win 5 Olympic gold medals (speed skating).
Also: **Bonny, Bunnie, Bunny.**

Boston: the name of the city used as a first name.

Brandy: popular modern name, after the liquor. Brandy, pop singer.
Also: **Brandi, Brandie.**

Bree: a form of Briana and other Bri- names. Breeda Bennehy, long-distance runner.

Brenda: (Celtic) "fiery."
Also: **Bren.**

Brenna: (Celtic) "maiden with black or raven hair."
Also: **Bren.**

Brett: *see* Brittany. Brett Butler, comedienne, actress.

Briana: (Gaelic) "strong." Feminine of Brian.
Also: **Breana, Bree, Breena, Brianna, Brianne, Brina, Brinn, Brynn, Brynne.**

Bridget: (Celtic) "mighty; strong." St. Bridget, patron saint of Sweden. Bridget Fonda, actress.
Also: **Birgit, Birgitta, Brieta, Brietta, Brigette, Brigida, Brigit, Brigitta, Brigitte, Brit, Brita.**

Brita: a form of Bridget.

Britt: (Scandinavian) "strong."
Also: **Brit.**

Brittany: (Latin) "from Britain"; a region in northwestern France.
Also: **Brett, Brit, Briton, Brittain, Brittan, Brittaney, Brittney.**

Bronte: (Greek) "thunder."

Bronwen: (Old Welsh) "white-bosomed."
Also: **Bronwyn.**

Brooke: (English) "brook; stream." Brooke Shields, actress.
Also: **Brook, Brooks.**

Brunhilde: (Teutonic) "heroine on the battlefield." Mythology: Brunhild was the leader of the Valkyries.
Also: **Brunhild, Brunhilda.**

Bryn: (Welsh) "hill."
Also: **Brynn, Brynne.**

Buena: (Spanish) "good."

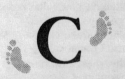

Cadence: (Latin) "rhythmic."
Also: **Cadenza.**

Cai: (Chinese) "cheer; prize; talent." Traditionally combined with another name. (Vietnamese) "female."

Caitlin: an Irish form of Catherine.
Also: **Catlin, Kaitlin, Kaitlyn.**

Calandra: (Greek) "lark."
Also: **Calandria, Calendre, Calley, Calli, Cally.**

Calantha: (Greek) "beautiful blossom."

Caledonia: (Latin) "from Scotland."

Caley: (Irish Gaelic) "thin, slender."

Calida: (Spanish) "warm, ardent."
Also: **Cali, Cally.**

California: (Spanish) the name of the Western state derived from the Greek meaning "beautiful sky."

Calista: (Greek) "most beautiful one"; Callisto is a satellite of the planet Jupiter.
Also: **Calla, Callista, Cally, Calysta, Kallista.**

Calla: (Greek) "beautiful"; also a flower name.
Also: **Calli, Callie, Cally.**

Callis: (Latin) "cup."

Callista: see Calista.

Callula: (Latin) "little beautiful one."

Callum: (Celtic) "dove." See also Columbia.

Cally: short form of names beginning Cal-.

Calypso: (Greek) Mythology: a sea nymph who held Odysseus captive on her island.

Cam: (Vietnamese) "the orange fruit"; also a short form of names beginning Cam-.

Camellia: a flower name. See also Camilla.

Cameo: (Italian) "a sculptured jewel."

Camera: from the word camera. Camera Ashe, daughter of Arthur Ashe, tennis great.

Cameron: (Celtic) "bent nose." Cameron Diaz, actress.
Also: **Cam.**

Camilla: (Latin) "noble; righ-teous." Legendary warrior maiden of Roman myth.
Also: **Cam, Camella, Camellia, Camille, Milla, Milly.**

Camille: see Camilla. Camille Gutt, head of the International Monetary Fund.

Campbell: (French) "from a bright field."
Also: **Cam.**

Canace: (Greek) "daughter of the wind."

Candace, Candice: (Latin) "pure; glowing fire-white." Candice Bergen, actress.
Also: **Candice, Candida, Candie, Candy, Kandace.**

Candida: see Candace. Candida Alvarez, painter.
Also: **Candide.**

Candra: (Latin) "luminous."

Candy: familiar form of Candace.

Canna: a botanical name.

Canyon: a contemporary name.

Caprice: (Italian) "fanciful."
Also: **Capricia.**

Cara: (Celtic) "friend."
Also: **Carah, Carrie, Kara.**

Caresse: (French) "endearing one."
Also: **Caressa.**

Cari: (Turkish) "flows like water."
Also: **Carrie.**

Carissa: see Charise.

Carita: (Latin) "beloved, dear one."

Carla: (Teutonic) "one who is strong." A feminine form of Charles.

Also: **Carley, Carlina, Carlita, Carly, Karla, Karli, Karly.**

Carleen: see Carol.

Carlotta: (Italian) "one who is strong." Another feminine form of Charles. See also Charlotte.

Carly: see Carla. Carly Simon, singer.

Carma: (Sanskrit) "fate; destiny."
Also: **Karma.**

Carmel: (Hebrew) "God's fruitful field." Biblical: Mount Carmel. Carmel Snow, fashion editor.
Also: **Carmela, Carmelina, Carmelita (Sp), Carmelle, Lita.**

Carmen: (Latin) "a song." (Spanish) "from Mount Carmel."
Also: **Carmel, Carmine.**

Carol: (French) "joyous song." Also a form of Charles.
Also: **Carey, Cari, Caril, Carleen, Carlene, Carline, Carly, Carola, Carole, Carolle, Carrie, Caryl, Karol.**

Caroline: (Teutonic) "one who is strong." Another feminine form of Charles. Carolyn Hershel, astronomer.
Also: **Carola, Carolina (It, Sp), Carolyn, Carrie, Karolina (Pol), Karoline, Karolyn, Lina.**

Caron: a French place name.

Carrie: see Carol, Caroline, Charlotte. Carrie Fisher, actress, writer.
Also: **Carey, Carie, Carre, Carry, Cary, Kari.**

Carson: the surname used as a first name. Carson McCullers, writer.

Carter: (Scottish) "cartmaker." Carter Heyward, one of the first group of female priests (b. 1945).

Casey: (Irish Gaelic) "brave."
Also: **Casie, Kacey, Kacie, Kasey.**

Cass, Cassie: short form of Cassandra, Cassidy.

Cassandra: (Greek) "the prophetess." Mythology: the daughter of Priam, king of Troy.
Also: **Casandra, Cass, Cassandre (Fr), Cassie, Cassy, Kassandra.**

Cassidy: (Irish) "curly-haired."

Cassiopeia: (Greek) "fragrance of roses." Mythology: Queen Cassiopeia, mother of the beautiful princess Andromeda.

Casta: (Latin) "pure, pious, modest one."

Catalina: Spanish form of Catherine.

Catherine: (Greek) "pure."
Also: **Catherina, Catherine, Cathleen, Kara, Karen, Karena, Karin, Karyn, Kat, Kate, Katharina, Kathe, Kathie, Kathleen, Kathlene, Kathryn, Kathy, Katie, Katrina, Katrine, Ketti, Kit, Kittie, Kitty, Trina.**

Cathi, Cathy: short forms of Catherine.

Cecilia, Cicely: (Latin) "musical." Feminine of Cecil. St. Cecilia, patroness of music and musicians. Cicely Tyson, actress.

Also: **Ceci, Cecile, Cecily, Celia, Cici, Cicily, Cis, Cissy.**

Celandine: (Greek) "the swallow."

Celeste: (Latin) "heavenly."
Also: **Celesta, Celestina, Celestine.**

Celia: *see* Cecilia. Celia Cruz, Latin singer.

Celine: a French form of Marcel. Celine Dion, singer. *See also* Selena.

Celosia: (Greek) "flaming, burning"; a flower name.

Cerelia: (Latin) "of the spring." Mythology: the Roman goddess of agriculture and grain.
Also: **Cerella.**

Cerise: (French) "cherry."
Also: **Cherry.**

Cezanne: a contemporary name inspired by the French Impressionist painter Paul Cezanne.

Chan: (Chinese) "lovely; the moon." Traditionally combined with another name.

Chandler: (French) "candlemaker."
Also: **Chan.**

Chandra: (Sanskrit) "she outshines the stars." Mythology: one of the names of the great Hindu goddess Shakti. Chandra Cheeseborough, Olympic gold medalist in track; Chanda Rubin, tennis player.

Chanel: (French) "channel."

Chaney: (Old French) "dweller at the oak forest." Chaney Holland, writer.

Chantal: (French) "a stone." The name honors St. Jeanne de Chantal, a 17th-century French saint. Chantal Akerman, film director.
Also: **Chantel, Chantelle, Shantal, Shantel, Shantelle.**

Chapin: (French) "a man of God."
Also: **Chapen, Chapland, Chaplin.**

Charis: *see* Charise.

Charise, Charissa: (Greek) "graceful."
Also: **Carissa, Charis.**

Charity: (Latin) "charitable; loving."
Also: **Charita, Cherry.**

Charlayne: a feminine form of Charles. Charlayne Hunter-Gault, television anchor.

Charlene, Charline: *see* Charlotte.

Charley: familiar form of Charlotte.

Charlotte: (Teutonic) "strong; womanly." Another feminine form of Charles. Charlotte Brontë, author; Charlotta Bass, editor.
Also: **Carlotta, Carrie, Carry, Charla, Charley, Charleen, Charlene, Charline, Letty, Lotta, Lotte, Lottie, Lotty.**

Charmaine: (Latin) "little song."
Also: **Charmain.** *See also* Carmen.

Chastity: (Latin) "purity."

Chastity Bono, daughter of Cher and Sonny Bono.

Chelsea: (English) "a port of ships"; a place name. Chelsea Clinton, daughter of U.S. President Bill Clinton.
Also: **Chelsey, Chelsie.**

Chen: (Chinese) "celestial bodies; treasure." Traditionally combined with another name. Chen Lu (Lu Chen), skater.

Chenoa: (American Indian) "white dove."

Cher: *see* Cherie. Cher, singer, actress.

Cherie: (French) "dear one."
Also: **Cher, Cherelle, Cheri, Cherice, Cherise, Cheryl, Sher, Sherilyn, Sherry, Sheryl.**

Cherry: (Old French) "cherrylike." Cherry Jones, Tony Award–winning actress.
Also: **Cherri.** *See also* Charise, Charity.

Cheryl: a form of Carol.

Chesna: (Slavic) "peaceful."
Also: **Chessy.**

Cheyenne: (French-Canadian Indian) name of an Algonquian tribe of the Great Plains.

Chiara: Italian form of Clara.

China, Chynna: contemporary place name. Chynna Phillips, singer/actress.

Chiquita: (Spanish) "little one."
Also: **Chicky.**

Chloe: (Greek) "fresh-blooming."
Also: **Chloette, Cloe.**

Chloris: (Greek) "pale flower."
Also: **Cloris.**

Chris: short form of Christine.

Christabel, Christabelle: *see* Christine.

Christiane: *see* Christine.

Christine: (Greek) "fair Christian." Feminine of Christian. Christina, queen of Sweden.
Also: **Chris, Chrissie, Chrissy, Christa, Christabel, Christabelle, Christal, Christiana, Christie, Christina, Christy, Chrystal, Crystal, Kirsten (Scand), Kirsty, Kris, Kristiana, Kristin, Kristina, Kristine, Krystyna, Teena, Tina.**

Ci: (Chinese) "loving." Traditionally combined with another name.

Cicily, Cis, Cissy: *see* Cecilia.

Cilla: a short form of Priscilla. Cilla Black, singer.

Cindy: *see* Cynthia, Lucinda.

Claire, Clare: *see* Clara.

Clara: (Latin) "bright; shining." Clara Barton, founder of the American Red Cross.
Also: **Chiara, Clair, Claire, Clarabelle, Clare, Clareta, Clarette, Clarinda, Clarine, Clarita, Klara.**

Clarabelle: combination of Clara and Belle.

Clarimond: (Old German) "bright protector."

Clarissa: (Latin-Greek) "one who will be famous."
Also: **Clarice, Clarisa, Clarise, Klarissa.**

Claudette: *see* Claudia.

Claudia: (Latin) "the lame." Feminine of Claud. Heroine of several novels by Colette.
Also: **Claude, Claudette, Claudie, Claudina, Claudine.**

Cleary: (Irish Gaelic) "scholar."

Clematis: (Greek) a flower name.

Clementine: (Greek) "merciful." Feminine of Clement. Mythology: Clementia was the Roman goddess of pity.
Also: **Clem, Clementina, Klementine.**

Cleo: (Greek) "of a famous father." Short form of Cleopatra. Cleo Laine, singer.

Cleopatra: (Greek) "of a famous father."
Also: **Cleo.**

Cleva: (Middle English) "dweller at the cliff."

Cliantha: (Greek) "glory-flower."

Clio: (Greek) "the proclaimer." Mythology: the Greek muse of history. *See also* Cleo.

Cloe: *see* Chloe.

Cloris: *see* Chloris.

Clotilde: (Teutonic) "famous battle maiden." French queen and saint.
Also: **Clothilde, Clotilda.**

Clover: (English) "clover blossom."

Clymene: (Greek) "renowned, famed one."
Also: **Clymenia.**

Cody: (English) "helpful."
Also: **Codi, Codie, Kody.**

Colette: (Greek-French) "victorious." Colette, French author.
Also: **Collett, Collette, Nicole, Nicolette.**

Colleen: (Irish) "girl." Colleen Dewhurst, actress.
Also: **Coleen, Colene.**

Columbia: (Latin) "the dove."
Also: **Callum, Columba.**

Columbine: a flower name.
Also: **Columbina.**

Comfort: (French) "strengthening aid and comfort." A Puritan name.

Conception: (Latin) "beginning." Conchita Martinez, tennis player.
Also: **Chita, Concepción, Concha, Concheta, Conchita.**

Concha: (Latin) "a shell." Concha Melendez, poet.

Concheta: a form of Conception.
Also: **Conchata.**

Concordia: (Latin) "harmony." Mythology: the goddess of peace after war.

Connie: a short form of Constance and other names beginning Con-. Connie Chung, broadcaster.

Connor: (Irish) "hound-lover."
Also: **Conner, Connie.**

Constance: (Latin) "constancy."
Also: **Connie, Constantia, Constantina, Constantine.**

Constant: a Puritan virtue name.

Consuela: (Latin) "consolation."
Also: **Connie, Consuelo.**

Cora: (Greek) "maiden."
Also: **Corabel, Corabelle, Corene, Coretta, Corette, Corinna, Corinne, Corita, Correna, Corrie, Corry.** *See also* Kora.

Coral: (Greek) "from the sea coral."
Also: **Coralie, Coraline, Koral.**

Corazon: (Spanish) "heart." Corazon Aquino, president of the Philippines.

Cordelia: (Celtic) "jewel of the sea."
Also: **Cordelie, Cordellia, Delia, Della.**

Coretta: a form of Cora. Coretta Scott King, civil rights leader.

Corinna, Corinne: a form of Cora. Mythology: Corinna was a Greek lyric poet.

Corita: *see* Cora. Corita Kent, artist.

Cornelia: (Latin) "horn-colored." Feminine of Cornelius.
Also: **Cornela, Nelia, Nell, Nellie.**

Cosima: (Greek) "order, harmony." The famed Cosima Wagner was the daughter of Franz Liszt and wife of Richard Wagner.

Courage: a Puritan virtue name.

Courtney: a French place name.
Also: **Cortney, Courtenay, Courtnay.**

Crescent: (Old French) "to increase or create."
Also: **Crescencia, Crescentia.**

Crystal, Crystele: *see* Christine. "clear as crystal." Crystele, model.
Also: **Christalle, Cristal, Crysta, Krystal.**

Cyanea: (Greek) "with eyes as blue as the sea."
Also: **Cyan.**

Cybil: a form of Sybil.

Cynara: (Greek) "thistle or artichoke."

Cynthia: (Greek) "moon." Cynthia Gregory, ballerina.
Also: **Cindy, Cyn, Cynth, Cynthea, Cynthie, Sindy, Synthia.**

Cyprien: (French) "from Cyprus." Cyprian, sister of Sylvia Beach, publisher.

Cypris: (Greek) "from the island of Cyprus."

Cyra: a form of Cyrena. Cyra McFadden, journalist and author.

Cyrena: (Greek) "from Cyrene."
Also: **Cyra, Cyrene.**

Cyrilla: a form of Cyrena.

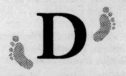

D

Dacia: (Greek) "from Dacia."
Also: **Dacey, Daci, Dacia, Dashia, Dasi.**

Daffodil: (Old French) "the daffodil flower."

Dahlia: (Scandinavian) "from the valley"; a flower name.
Also: **Dalia.**

Daisy: (Anglo-Saxon) "the day's eye."
Also: **Daisie.**

Dakota: (American Indian—Sioux) "alliance of friends."

Dale: (Teutonic) "dweller in the valley." Dayle Haddon, model.
Also: **Dail, Daile.**

Dalila: (Swahili) "a sign."
Also: **Lila.**

Dallas: (Gaelic) "from the dales"; the place name used as a first name for both boys and girls.

Damara: (Greek) "gentle girl."
Also: **Damaris, Mara.**

Damita: (Spanish) "little noble lady."

Dana: (Scandinavian) "from Denmark."

Danae: (Greek) Mythology: the mother of Perseus.
Also: **Danella, Denae.**

Danica: (Old Slavic) "morning star."
Also: **Danika.**

Danielle: (Hebrew/French) "judged by God." Feminine form of Daniel.
Also: **Danella, Danelle, Dani, Daniela, Daniele, Danila, Danita, Danni, Dannie, Danny.**

Daphne: (Greek) "laurel tree." Mythology: the nymph who, when pursued by Apollo, was transformed into a laurel tree.
Also: **Daffy, Daph, Daphie.**

Dara: (Hebrew) "compassion."
Also: **Darah.**

Darcie: (French-Celtic) "from the stronghold; dark one." Darci Kirstler, ballerina.
Also: **Dara, Darcy.**

Darice: (Persian) "queenlike."
Also: **Dareece, Darees, Dari, Daria.**

Darlene: (Anglo-Saxon) "dearly beloved."
Also: **Darleen, Darline, Daryl.**

Daron: (Irish Gaelic) Feminine form of Darren.

Daryl: see Darlene. Daryl Hannah, actress.
Also: **Darryl.**

Dascha: (Greek) "gift of God."
Also: **Dasha.**

Davida: Feminine of David.
Also: **Davina, Davita.**

Davina: (Hebrew) "the loved." Feminine of David.
Also: **Davida, Davita.**

Dawn: (Anglo-Saxon) "the break of day."

Deandra: combination of Deanna and Sandra.

Deanna: a form of Diana.
Also: **Deana, Deanne.**

Deborah: (Hebrew) "the bee." Biblical: the great Hebrew prophetess.
Also: **Deb, Debbi, Debbie, Debby, Debi, Debora.**

Debra: see Deborah.

Dee: see Audrey, Deidre, Dorothy.

Deidre: (Gaelic) "sorrow."

Deidre Hall, soap opera star.
Also: **Dee, Deedee, Deirdre, Didi, Dierdre.**

Delfina: *see* Delphine.

Delia: (Greek) "from the isle of Delos." Delia Ephron, writer.
Also: **Dede, Dee, Della.** *See also* Cordelia.

Delicia: (Latin) "delightful one."
Also: **Delight, Delisha, Delizia.**

Delilah: (Hebrew) "the temptress." Biblical: the mistress of Samson.
Also: **Dalila, Delila, Lila, Lilah.**

Della: (Teutonic) "noble." Della Reese, singer.
Also: **Del.** *See also* Adelaide, Cordelia.

Delphine: (Greek) "dolphin; the delphinium flower."
Also: **Delfine, Delphina.**

Delta: (Greek) fourth letter of the Greek alphabet.

Delyth: (Welsh) "pretty."
Also: **Del.**

Demetria: (Greek) "from a fertile land." Mythology: Demeter, Greek goddess of the harvest. Demi Moore, actress.
Also: **Demi, Demitria, Demy, Dimitria.**

Dena: (Old English) "from the valley." Feminine of Dean.
Also: **Deana, Deane, Deanna, Denni, Dina.**

Denae: *see* Danae.

Denise, Denyce: (Greek) "wine goddess." Feminine

of Dennis. Denyce Graves, opera singer.
Also: **Denice, Denny, Denys.**

Denver: (Old English) "dweller at the valley edge"; the place name.

Dervla: (Irish) "true desire." Dervla Murphy, Irish adventurer.
Also: **Devilia.**

Desdemona: (Greek) "girl of sadness." Literary: wife of Shakespeare's Othello.
Also: **Demona, Desdamona, Mona.**

Desiree: (Latin-French) "desired."
Also: **Desirata, Desiray.**

Desma: (Greek) "a bond or pledge."

Deva: (Sanskrit) "divine." Mythology: the goddess of the moon.

Devin: *see* Devon.

Devlin: (Irish Gaelic) "fierce valor."

Devon: (Old English) "from Devonshire."
Also: **Devin, Devona.**

Devotion: a Puritan virtue name.

Dextra: (Latin) "skillful, dexterous." Feminine of Dexter.

Diamantha: (French) "diamondlike."
Also: **Diamond.**

Diana: In Roman myth, the goddess of the hunt and chaste goddess of the moon. Dian Fossey, primatologist.
Also: **Deanna, Di, Diane, Dianna, Dyan.** *See also* Deanna.

Diane: *see* Diana. Diane Arbus, photographer.

Diantha: "flower of Zeus; divine flower."
Also: **Dianthe.**

Dierdre: *see* Deidre.

Dilys: (Welsh) "genuine."
Also: **Dil.**

Dina: *see* Dinah.

Dinah: (Hebrew) "judged; exonerated." Biblical: daughter of Jacob and Leah. Dinah Shore, singer.
Also: **Dina, Dynah.**

Dione: (Greek) "the daughter of heaven and earth." Mythology: the mother of Aphrodite. Dionne Warwick, singer.
Also: **Dion, Dionne.**

Disa: (Old Norse) "active sprite."

Dixie: (French) "ten, tenth." From the name for the American South. Dixy Lee Ray, first woman governor of Washington, scientist.
Also: **Dixy.**

Dodi: *see* Doris.

Doe: (English) "the doe or female deer." Doe Avedon, actress.

Dolley, Dollie, Dolly: *see* Dorothy. Dolley Madison, First Lady of the U.S.

Dolores: (Latin) "our lady of sorrows."
Also: **Delora, Delores, Deloris, Dori, Dorrie, Dorry, Lola.**

Domina: (Latin) "lady."

Dominica: (Latin) "born on the Lord's day." Feminine of Dominic.
Also: **Dominee, Dominga, Dominique (Fr).**

Dominique: *see* Dominica.

Donata: (Latin) "donation; gift."

Donna: (Italian) "lady."
Also: **Dona, Donella, Donelle.**

Dora: (Greek) "a gift." *See also* Dorothy, Eudora, Isadora.

Dore: (French) "golden one."

Dorene: (French) "golden."
Also: **Doreen, Dori, Dorie, Dorine, Dorrie, Dorry.**

Dori, Dorie, Dorrie, Dorry: *see* Delores, Dorene, Dorinda, Isadora, Pandora, Theodora.

Dorinda: a form of Dora.
Also: **Dori, Dorin.**

Doris: (Greek) "sea goddess." Mythology: the Greek sea goddess. Doris Lessing, author.
Also: **Dodi.**

Dorothy: (Greek) "God's gift." A feminine form of Theodore. Dorothea Dix, 19th-century activist for the mentally ill.
Also: **Dee, Dollie, Dolly, Dora, Dore, Doretta, Dorotea, Dorothea, Dorothi, Dorthea, Dorthy, Dot, Dottie, Dotty.**

Dottie, Dotty: *see* Dorothy. Dottie Mochrie, golfer.

Dover: (English) "from Dover."

Drew: a form of Andrew. Drew Barrymore, actress.

Druella: (Old German) "elfin vision."

Drusilla: (Greek) "soft-eyed."
Also: **Dru, Drucilla.**

Duana: (Irish Gaelic) "little dark one."

Duena: (Spanish) "chaperone."

Dulcinea: (Latin) "charming; sweet."
Also: **Dulci, Dulcia, Dulcie, Dulcine.**

Durra: (Swahili) "pearl."
Also: **Durah.**

Dusty: a feminine form of Dustin. Dusty Springfield, singer.

Dyan: variant of Diane. Dyan Cannon, actress, filmmaker.

Dylan: (Welsh) "from the sea."
Also: **Dillon, Dylane.**

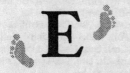

Earlene: (Old English) "noble woman." Feminine of Earl.
Also: **Earla, Earline.**

Eartha: (Old English) "of the earth." Eartha Kitt, singer.
Also: **Erda, Ertha, Herta.**

Ebba: (Old English) "flowing back of the tide."

Ebony: (Greek) the rare, prized black wood.
Also: **Ebonie.**

Ebrilla: a Welsh form of April.

Echo: (Greek) "reflected sound." Mythology: the Greek nymph whose speech was taken away by the jealous goddess Hera.

Eda: (Old English) "prosperity, blessedness."
Also: **Ede.**

Edana: (Irish-Gaelic) "little fiery one."

Ede: *see* Eda.

Eden: (Hebrew) "enchanting"; the Biblical place name.
Also: **Edena.**

Edie: *see* Edith.

Edina: (Scotch) "from the city of Edinburgh."

Edita: Spanish form of Edith.
Also: **Edyta (Pol).**

Edith: (Teutonic) "rich gift." Edith Wharton, novelist.
Also: **Eadie, Eadith, Eda, Ede, Edie, Edina, Edita, Editha, Edithe, Edyta (Pol), Edythe.**

Edlyn: (Anglo-Saxon) "of nobility."
Also: **Lyn.**

Edmonda: (Old English) feminine of Edmund.

Edmonia: *see* Edmonda. Edmonia Lewis, sculptor.

Edna: (Hebrew) "rejuvenation." Edna Ferber, author.
Also: **Edie, Ednah, Edny.** *See also* Ada.

Edrea: (Old English) "prosperous, powerful."
Also: **Edra.**

Edwina: (Anglo-Saxon) "valued friend." A feminine form of Edwin.
Also: **Edwine, Win, Wina, Winnie, Winny.**

Effie: (Greek) "fair and famed."
Also: **Effy.** *See also* Euphemia.

Eileen: *see* Aileen.

Eira: (Welsh) "snow."
Also: **Eiry.**

Eirene: (Greek) "peace."
Also: **Eir, Eirena.**

Eirlys: (Welsh) "snowdrop."
Eirlys Roberts, English consumer activist.

Eirwen: (Welsh) "snow-white."

Ekaterina: Russian form of Catherine. Ecaterina Szabo, Romanian gymnast.

Elaine: (Greek) "light."
Also: **Alaine, Alayne, Elaina, Elana, Elane, Elayne, Laine.**

Elata: (Latin) "lofty, elevated."

Elberta: *see* Alberta.

Eldora: (Spanish) "gilded one."
Also: **Eldoria.**

Eleanor: A form of Helen. Eleanor of Aquitaine; Eleanor Roosevelt, First Lady, social activist.
Also: **Eleanora, Eleanore, Elenore, Elinor, Elinore, Ellie, Lena, Lenora, Leonora.**

Electra: (Greek) "shining star." Mythology: the daughter of Agamemnon, king of Mycenae and Clytemnestra.
Also: **Lectra.**

Elena: a form of Eleanor, Helen.
Also: **Eleni (Greek).**

Eleri: (Welsh) the name of a female 5th-century Welsh saint.

Elexa: *see* Alexandra.

Elfreda: (Teutonic) "noble and wise." Feminine of Albert.
Also: **Elfrida, Elfrieda.**

Elga: (Slavic) "holy, consecrated."

Elise: a French form of Elizabeth. *See also* Elysia.

Elissa: *see* Elizabeth. Mythology: Dido (Elissa) was the queen of Carthage.

Elita: (Latin) "select; a special person."
Also: **Lita.**

Eliza: *see* Elizabeth. Eliza Doolittle, of George Bernard Shaw's *Pygmalion* (1914).

Elizabeth: (Hebrew) "consecrated to God." Biblical: the mother of John the Baptist.
Also: **Bess, Bessie, Beth, Betsy, Betsey, Bette, Betti, Bettina (It), Betty, Elisa, Elisabeth, Elisabetta (It), Elise (Fr), Eliza, Elsa, Elsbeth, Else, Elsie, Elzbieta (Pol), Isabel (Sp), Libby, Liesl (Ger), Lisa, Lisabet, Lisabeth, Lisbeth, Lise, Liz, Liza, Lizzie, Lizzy, Ysabel.**

Elke: a Germanic form of Alice. Elkie Brooks, British rock singer.

Ella, Ellie: *see* Helen. Ella Fitzgerald, singer; Ella Grasso, governor of Connecticut.

Ellamay: combination of Ella and May.
Also: **Ellamae.**

Elle: (French) the personal pronoun "she." Elle Macpherson, model.

Ellen: a form of Helen.
Also: **Elena, Ellie, Elly, Ellyn.**

Ellice: (Greek) feminine of Elias.

Elma: (Greek) "pleasant."

Elmira: *see* Almira.

Elodie: (Greek) "marsh flower."

Eloise: a French form of Louise.
Also: **Eloisa.**

Elsa, Elsie: *see* Elizabeth. Elsa Lanchester, actress.

Elvina: (Old English) "elfin friend."

Elvira: (Spanish) "like an elf."
Also: **Elva, Elvera, Elvie.**

Elysia: (Latin) "sweetly blissful." In Roman mythology, Elysium is the abode of happy souls.
Also: **Elicia, Elise, Elisha, Elyse, Ilyse.**

Emblem: a form of Amelia.

Emeline: *see* Emmeline.

Emerald: (Old French) the green gemstone.
Also: **Emeraude.**

Emi: (EH-mee) (Japanese) "blessed; beautiful."
Also: **Emiko.**

Emilia: *see* Emily.

Emily: (Teutonic) "industrious." A feminine form of Emil. Emily Dickinson, poet; Emily Balch, winner of the Nobel Peace Prize.
Also: **Em, Emelda, Emilia, Emilie, Emlyn, Emmy, Millie.**
See also Amelia.

Emlyn: a Welsh place name.

Emma: (Teutonic) "one who heals." Emma Bovary, the most famous heroine in 19th-century French fiction.
Also: **Em, Emeline, Emelyne, Emie, Emmaline, Emmie, Emmy.**

Emmanuelle: (Hebrew/French) "God is with us." Feminine of Emanuel.

Emmeline: *see* Amelia. Emmeline Pankhurst (1858–1928), who secured the vote for British women.

Emmylou: combination of Emma and Louise. Emmylou Harris, country singer.

Ena: (Irish Gaelic) "little ardent or fiery one."

Endora: (Hebrew) "fountain."

Enid: (Celtic) "purity of soul." Enid Bagnold, British novelist.

Ennea: (Greek) "wine."

Enola: (English) an American name that gained notoriety when the U.S. bomber Enola Gay, named after the captain's mother, dropped the atom bomb on Hiroshima in 1945.

Enrica: *see* Henrietta.

Eolande: *see* Yolande.

Epifania: (German/Spanish) "the Epiphany."

Erda: *see* Hertha.

Erica: (Scandinavian) "of royalty." Feminine of Eric. Erica Jong, writer.
Also: **Erika, Rica, Ricky, Rika, Riki.**

Erin: (Celtic) "girl from Ireland."
Also: **Erina, Eryn.**

Erlinda: (Hebrew) "lively." Erlinda Gonzales-Berry, educator.

Erma: *see* Irma.

Ernestine: (Teutonic) "earnest; purposeful; token of the eagle." Feminine of Ernest.
Also: **Erna, Ernesta, Ernestina, Teena, Tina.**

Erselia: (Latin) meaning unclear.
Also: **Ersilia, Hersilia.**

Ertha: *see* Eartha.

Erwina: (Old English) "friend." Feminine of Erwin.

Esme: (French) "esteemed."
Also: **Esmee.**

Esmeralda: (Greek/Spanish) "emerald."
Also: **Emerald, Esme, Ezmeralda, Merald.**

Esperanza: (Spanish) "hope."

Esta: (Italian) "from the east." *See also* Vesta.

Estelle, Estelita: (Latin) "a star." Estelita Rodriguez, actress.
Also: **Estela, Estella, Estrelita, Estrella (Sp), Stella.**

Esther: (Hebrew) "a star." Biblical: the queen of Persia.
Also: **Essie, Essy, Esta, Ester, Hester, Hettie, Hetty.**

Ethel: (Teutonic) "noble."
Also: **Ethyl.**

Ethelind, Etheline, Ethelyn: forms of Ethel.

Etheljean: (Teutonic) "noble with divine grace."

Ethlyne: a form of Ethel.

Etsuko: (et-SOO-koh) (Japanese) "rejoice, child."
Also: **Ets.**

Etta: *see* Henrietta. Etta James, rhythm and blues singer.

Euclea: (Greek) "glory."

Eudocia: (Greek) "esteemed."
Also: **Docia, Eudosia.**

Eudora: (Greek) "wonderful gift." Eudora Welty, author.
Also: **Dora.**

Eugenia: (Greek) "wellborn." Feminine of Eugene. Eugenie, empress of France.
Also: **Eugenie, Gena, Gene, Genie, Gina.**

Eulalia: (Greek) "fair speech; well-spoken one."
Also: **Eula, Eulalie, Lallie.**

Eunice: (Greek) "gloriously victorious."

Euphemia: (Greek) "fair and famed."
Also: **Effie, Effy, Euphemie.**

Eustacia: (Latin) "stable, tranquil." Feminine of Eustace.
Also: **Stace, Stacie, Stacy.**

Eva: *see* Eve.

Evadne: (Greek) "fortunate." Mythology: the daughter of Poseidon and Pitana, loved by Apollo.

Evangeline: (Greek) "bearer of good news." Evangeline Booth, first woman commander of the Salvation Army.
Also: **Eva, Evangelina, Evangelista (It), Eve.**

Eve: (Hebrew) "life; living." Biblical: Eve the first woman, mother of Cain, Abel, and Seth.
Also: **Eva, Eveleen, Evelina,**

Eveline, Evelyn, Evie, Evita, Evonne, Ewa (Pol).

Evelyn: *see* Eve.

Evonne: *see* Eve. Evonne Goolagong, tennis player.

Ewa: (Polish) "life." Ewa Mataya, pool player.

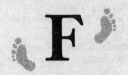

Fabiana: (Latin) "bean grower." Feminine of Fabian.
Also: **Fabia, Fabianna, Fabianne, Favianna.**

Fabiola: *see* Fabiana. Fabiola Cabeza de Baca Gilbert, home economist, author.

Fae: a form of Fay.

Faida: (Icelandic) "winged."

Faith: (Latin) "trusting; faithful." Faith Hill, country singer.
Also: **Fae, Fay, Faye.**

Faline: (Latin) "catlike."

Fallon: (Irish Gaelic) "of a ruling family."
Also: **Faline, Falyn.**

Fanchette: (French) "little free one."

Fanchon: (French) "free."

Fanny: *see* Frances. Fanny Farmer, cookbook author; Fannia Mary Cohn, labor leader.
Also: **Fan, Fannie.**

Farida: (Arabic) "unique."

Farrah: (Arabic) "happy." Farrah Fawcett, actress.

Fatima: (Arabic) a daughter of the prophet Mohammed.
Also: **Fatuma.**

Faustina: (Latin) "lucky."
Also: **Faustena, Faustine.**

Favianna: *see* Fabiana.

Favonia: (Latin) "the West Wind."

Favor: (Old French) "help, approval."

Fawn: (Old French) "young deer; reddish-brown."
Also: **Fanya, Faun, Fawne, Fawnia.**

Fay, Faye: (Old French) "fairy"; a form of Faith.
Also: **Fae.**

Fayanne: combination of Fay and Anne.

Fayette: (Old French) "little fairy."

Fayme: (Old French) "lofty reputation."

Fealty: (Old French) "fidelity, allegiance."
Also: **Feala.**

Felda: (Old German) "from the field."

Felicia: (Latin) "happiness." Feminine of Felix.
Also: **Felice, Felicity, Felise.**

Felicity: (Latin) the Roman goddess of happiness or good fortune.
Also: **Felicite (Fr).** *See also* Felicia.

Fenella: (Irish Gaelic) "white-shouldered one."
Also: **Finella.**

Feodora: (Greek) "God's gift." Feminine of Theodore.

Ferelith: (Celtic) "perfect princess."

Fern: (English) a plant name.

Fernanda: (German) "adventurer." Feminine of Ferdinand.
Also: **Ferdinanda, Fernandina.**

Feronia: (Latin) In Roman mythology, a goddess presiding over groves and forests.

Fidelity: (Latin) "faithful."
Also: **Fidela, Fidelia, Fidella.**

Fifi: *see* Josephine.

Filipa: *see* Philippa.

Filma: (Old English) "a veil or mist."

Finley: (Irish) "little fair-haired valorous one."
Also: **Findlay.**

Fionna: (Celtic) "ivory-skinned."
Also: **Fiona, Phiona, Viona, Vionna.**

Flanna: (Irish-Gaelic) "red-haired."
Also: **Flan.**

Flannery: (Old French) "a flat piece of metal." Flannery O'Connor, American writer. (1925–1964).
Also: **Flan.**

Flavia: (Latin) "yellow-haired; blond."

Fleta: (Old English) "swift, fleet one."

Fleur: (French) "flower."
Also: **Fleurette.**

Flora: (Latin) "flower." The Roman goddess of flowers.
Also: **Fiorenza (It), Florette (Fr),** Floria, Florida (Sp), Florenza, Floris.

Florence: (Latin) "to flower and bloom." Florence Nightingale, founder of modern nursing (1820–1910).
Also: **Fleur, Fleurette, Flo, Flora, Florentina, Florentyna, Florenza, Florette, Floria, Florine, Floris, Florrie, Flossie, Flower.**

Florida: (Latin) "flowery, blooming." A Spanish form of Florence.

Flower: (French) "a blossom." *See also* Florence.

Fonda: (Middle English) "affectionate; tender."

Fontana: (Italian) "dweller near the spring."

Fortune: (Latin) "fate, destiny."
Also: **Fortuna, Fortunata.**

Frances: (Latin) "free." Feminine of Francis. Frances Perkins, the first woman cabinet member in U.S. history (1933).
Also: **Fanny, Fran, Franca, France, Francesca, Francine, Frankie, Franky, Franny.**

Francesca: *see* Frances.

Freda: (Teutonic) "peace." A feminine form of Frederick.
Also: **Fredie, Freida, Frida, Frieda.** *See also* Wilfreda.

Fredella: contemporary name combining Freda and Ella.

Frederica: (Teutonic) "peaceful." Feminine form of Frederick.
Also: **Freddie, Freddy,**

Frederika, Frederique, Fredrika, Ricky. *See also* Freda.

Freya: (Scandinavian) the Norse goddess of fertility, famous for her beauty.

Frieda: *see* Freda. Frida Kahlo, Mexican artist.

Fritzie: (Teutonic) "peaceful ruler." Feminine of Fritz. Also: **Fritzi, Fritzy.**

Fronde: (Latin) "a leafy branch."

Fuji: (FOO-gee) (Japanese) "wisteria."

Fulvia: (Latin) "tawny or golden."

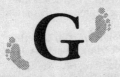

Gabey, Gabie: *see* Gabrielle.

Gabina: *see* Gavina.

Gabriela: a form of Gabrielle. Gabriela Sabatini, tennis player.

Gabrielle: (Hebrew) "woman of God." Feminine of Gabriel.
Also: **Gabey, Gabi, Gabie, Gabriela, Gabriella, Gaby.**

Gaea: (Greek) "the earth." Mythology: the Greek goddess of the earth.

Gail: short form of Abigail.
Also: **Gael, Gale, Gayle.**

Galatea: (Greek) "milky white." Mythology: the statue brought to life by

Aphrodite for Pygmalion, the sculptor, who had fallen in love with his creation.

Gale: *see* Abigail.

Galina: a Russian form of Helen. Galina Ulanova, ballerina.

Gardenia: (Latin) the fragrant white flower.

Garland: (Old French) "a wreath of flowers."
Also: **Garlande.**

Garnet: (Teutonic) "the red gemstone."
Also: **Garnette.**

Gavina: (Latin) "from Gabio."
Also: **Gabina.**

Gaviota: (Spanish) "seagull."

Gavrila: (Hebrew) "hero." A feminine form of Gabriel.

Gay: (Old French) "merry."
Also: **Gae, Gaye.**

Gazella: (Latin) "gazelle or antelope."
Also: **Gazelle.**

Gelasia: (Greek) "inclined to laughter."

Gelsey: origin and meaning uncertain. Gelsey Kirkland, ballerina.

Gemini: (Greek) "twin."
Also: **Gemina.**

Gemma: (Italian) "a gem or precious stone."
Also: **Gema, Jemma.**

Gena, Gene: a form of Jean. *See also* Eugenia, Regina.

Genara: (Latin) "born in the first month."

Genessa: (Hebrew) "origin."
Also: **Genesis, Genisia.**

Geneva: a form of Genevieve; the Swiss place name.
Also: **Geneve.**

Genevieve: (German) "white; pure." Genevieve (c.422–512), the patron saint of Paris; Genevieve Rose Cline, first woman appointed a U.S. federal judge.
Also: **Gena, Geneva, Gennie, Genny, Jennie, Jenny.**

Gentian: (Greek) a flower name.

Georgette: *see* Georgia.

Georgia: (Greek) "farmer." Feminine of George. Georgia O'Keeffe, artist.
Also: **Georgetta, Georgette, Georgi, Georgiana, Georgie, Georgina, Georgine.**

Georgiana: *see* Georgia. Georgiana Roberton, model.

Geraldine: (Teutonic) "ruler with a spear." Feminine of Gerald. Geraldine Ferraro, former congresswoman and vice presidential candidate.
Also: **Geralda, Geri, Gerri, Gerry, Jeraldine, Jerri, Jerrie, Jerry.**

Geranium: (Greek) the flower.

Gerda: (Teutonic) "the protected."
Also: **Garda, Gerdi.**

Germain: (French) "a German." Germaine Greer, author.

Germana: (German) "warrior."

Gertrude: (Teutonic) "spear maiden." Gerty Cori, first American woman to win the Nobel Prize for medicine and physiology; Gertrude Jekyll, garden designer (1843–1932).
Also: **Gerta, Gerti, Gertie, Gertrudis, Gerty, Trude, Trudy.**

Ghislaine: (Old German) "pledge." A form of Giselle.

Ghita: a familiar form of Margharita.

Giacinta: (Greek) "dark flower." *See also* Hyacinth, Jacinda.

Gianna: Italian form of Jane.
Also: **Gia, Giana.**

Gigi: (French) familiar form of Gabrielle. Gigi Fernandez, tennis player.

Gilberta: (Teutonic) "the bright pledge." Feminine of Gilbert.
Also: **Berta, Gil, Gilberte, Gilbertina, Gilbertine, Gilly.**

Gilda: (English) "gilded." Gilda Radner, comedienne.
Also: **Gilli.**

Gillian: (Latin) "youthful, downy-haired one." Gillian Armstrong, film director.
Also: **Gill, Gilliane, Jillian.**

Gina: *see* Angela, Eugenia, Regina. Geena Davis, actress.

Ginger: (English) the spice or flower. *See also* Virginia.

Giordana: Italian form of Jordan.

Giovanna: (Italian) feminine form of John.

Giselle: (French) "a promise." *Giselle,* the ballet.
Also: **Ghislaine, Gisela (Sp), Gisele, Gizela, Jiselle.**

Gita: (Hindi) "song."
Also: **Ghita.**

Gitta: (Hebrew) "goodness."

Giuliana: Italian form of Julia.
Giuliana Benetton, Italian
designer, businesswoman.

Gladys: (Latin) "frail; delicate;
the gladiolus flower." Also a
Welsh form of Claudia.
Also: **Glad, Gladdie, Gladine,
Gladis.**

Glenda: see Glenna.

Glendine: see Glenna.

Glenna: (Irish Gaelic) "from
the valley." Feminine of
Glenn. Glenn Close, actress.
Also: **Glen, Glenda, Glendine,
Glennie, Glennis, Glynis,
Glynnis.**

Gloria: (Latin) "glory." Gloria
Steinem, feminist, editor.
Also: **Glori, Glory.**

Gloriana: combination of
Gloria and Anna; thus, "glo-
rious grace."
Also: **Glorianna.**

Glynis, Glynnis: see Glenna.

Golda: (Old English) "the
golden one." Golda Meir,
prime minister of Israel
(1898–1978); Goldie Hawn,
actress.
Also: **Goldy.**

Goldie: see Golda.

Gordon: (Anglo-Saxon) "from
the cornered hill." Gordon
Hamilton, social work educator.

Grace: (Latin) "graceful."
Also: **Gracia (Sp), Gracie,
Graciela, Gracye, Grazia (It).**

Gracia: see Grace.

Gracienne: (Latin) "graceful
one."

Grayson: (Old English) "a
judge's son." Grayson Hall,
actress.
Also: **Graydon, Greyson.**

Grazia: variant of Grace.
Grazia Deledda, Nobel
prize–winning author.

Graziella: see Grace.

Gredel, Greta, Gretchen: see
Margaret. Grete Waitz, mar-
athon champion.

Greer: (Scottish) "the
watchwoman." Greer Gar-
son, actress.

Gregoria: (Latin) "watchful
one."

Griselda: (Teutonic) "the her-
oine."
Also: **Grissel, Grizella, Selda,
Zelda.**

Guadalupe: (Arabic) "valley
of the wolf." Guadalupe,
the patron saint of Mexico.
Also: **Lupe.**

Gudrun: (Teutonic) "God;
wisdom." A character in the
D. H. Lawrence novel
Women in Love.

Guenevere: see Guinevere.

Guenna: a short form of
Guenevere.

Guida: (Italian) "a guide."

Guinevere, Guenevere:
(Celtic) "fair lady."
Guenevere, wife of King Ar-
thur.
Also: **Gen, Genny, Guenevere,
Jen, Jenni, Jennie, Jennifer,
Jenny.**

Gusta: see Augusta.

Gwendolen: (Celtic) "white-

browed." Gwendolyn Brooks, Pulitzer prize–winning poet.
Also: **Gwen, Gwendolyn, Gwenn, Gwyn, Gwyneth.**

Gweneth, Gwyneth: (Welsh) "blessed." Gwyneth Paltrow, actress.
Also: **Gwenith.**

Gwynne: (Welsh) "fair one."

Gyda: (Teutonic) "gift."

Gypsy: (Old English) "wanderer."

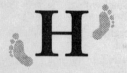

Habiba: (Arabic/Swahili) "beloved."

Hadara: (Hebrew) "beautiful."

Hadassah: (Hebrew) "myrtle." Hadassah, the Women's Zionist Organization of America.

Hadley: (English) "field of heather."

Hagar: (Hebrew) "one who flees." Biblical: the maid of Sarah, wife of Abraham. Hagar bore Abraham's son Ismael.
Also: **Haggar.**

Hahn: (Vietnamese) "faithful, moral."

Haidee: (Greek) "modest; honored."
Also: **Haide, Haydee.**

Haima: (Sanskrit) "golden."

Halcyone: (Greek) "sea-conceived." Mythology: grief-stricken over the death of her husband, Ceyx, Halcyone leaped into the sea, where she and her husband were transformed into kingfishers. Halcyone Bohen, Princeton's first woman dean.
Also: **Halcie.**

Haldana: (Old Norse) "half Danish."

Haley: (English) "hay meadow."
Also: **Hayley.**

Halima: (Arabic/Swahili) "gentle."
Also: **Halime.**

Hallie: (English) "from the hall." Hallie Flanagan, director of the Federal Theatre Project.
Also: **Hali, Halley, Halli, Hally.**
See also Hayley.

Halona: (American Indian) "happy fortune."

Hamelia: (Latin) a small genus of tropical shrubs which bear brilliant flowers.

Hana: (HAH-na) (Japanese) "flower."
Also: **Hanako.**

Hanani: variant of Hannah.
Also: **Hananiah.**

Hanley: (Anglo-Saxon) "of the high meadow."
Also: **Hanleigh, Henleigh, Henley, Henry.**

Hannabell: (Hebrew-French) "graceful beauty."

Hannah: (Hebrew) "full of grace, mercy, and prayer." Biblical: the mother of Sam-

uel. Hannah Arendt, philosopher; Hanna Gray, president of the University of Chicago.
Also: **Ann, Anna, Hanna, Hannie, Hanny.** *See also* Ann.

Hannette: (Hebrew) "little graceful one."

Happy: a contemporary name; "a happy child; joyful." Happy Rockefeller, wife of U.S. Vice President Nelson Rockefeller.

Haralda: feminine of Harold.

Harmony: (Latin) "concord, harmony."
Also: **Harmonia.**

Harper: (Old English) "harp player." Harper Lee, author of *To Kill a Mockingbird.*

Harriet: (Teutonic) "mistress of the home." Feminine of Henry. Harriet Tubman, abolitionist; Harriet Beecher Stowe, writer.
Also: **Harrietta, Harriette, Hatti, Hattie, Hatty.**

Haru: (HAR-oo) (Japanese) "spring."

Hattie, Hatty: *see* Harriet. Hattie Wyatt Caraway, first woman elected to the U.S. Senate (1932).

Haven: (English) "place of refuge."

Hayley: (English) "hay meadow."
Also: **Haley.**

Hazel, Hazelle: (Anglo-Saxon) the hazel tree. Hazel Brannon Smith, first woman to win the Pulitzer prize for editorial writing (1984);

Hazelle Goodman, comedienne.

Heather: (Anglo-Saxon) an evergreen flowering plant.
Also: **Heath.**

Hedda: (Teutonic) "war." The title character in Henrik Ibsen's play *Hedda Gabler.*
Also: **Heddy, Hedy.**

Heidi: *see* Hilda.

Helen: (Greek) "light." St. Helena, mother of the Emperor Constantine. Mythology: the beautiful wife of the Spartan king Menelaus, whose abduction by Paris is said to have sparked the Trojan War.
Also: **Eleanor, Eleanora, Eleanore, Elena, Elene, Elenore, Elinor, Elinore, Ella, Ellen, Ellie, Elnore, Helaina, Helena, Helene, Hellene, Lena, Lenni, Lennie, Lenore, Leonora, Leonore, Leora, Lora, Lorine, Nell, Nellie, Nelly, Nora, Yelena.**

Helena: *see* Helen. Helena Rubinstein, entrepreneur.

Helga: (Teutonic) "holy."

Helia: (Greek) "sun."

Helice: (Greek) "special."
Also: **Helise.**

Helma: (Old German) "helmet; protection."

Heloise: *see* Louise.

Helsa: (Hebrew) "given to God."

Hendrika: *see* Henrietta.

Henni, Hennie: *see* Henrietta.

Henrietta: (Teutonic) "mistress of the home." Feminine

form of Henry. Hetty (Henrietta) Green, financier.
Also: **Enrica, Etta, Etty, Hattie, Hendrika, Henni, Hennie, Henriette, Henrika, Henryka (Pol), Hetti, Hetty.**

Henrika: *see* Henrietta.

Hera: queen of the Olympian gods.

Herlinda: (Teutonic) "heroic beauty."
Also: **Erlinda.**

Hermina: *see* Hermione.

Hermione: (Greek) "of the earth." Feminine of Herman. Mythology: the daughter of Helen of Troy and Menelaus.
Also: **Erma, Hermina, Herminia.**

Hermosa: (Spanish) "beautiful."

Hersilia: *see* Erselia.

Hertha: (Teutonic) "earth mother." Hertha Ayrton, British inventor, physicist (1854–1923).
Also: **Eartha, Erda, Herta.**

Hesper: (Greek) "night star."

Hester: (Greek) "star." Hester Prynne, heroine of Hawthorne's *The Scarlet Letter* (1850).
Also: **Hetti, Hettie, Hetty.** *See also* Esther.

Hetti, Hettie Hetty: familiar forms of Henrietta, Hester. Hetty Goldman, the first woman to direct an archaeological excavation (1911).

Hilary: (Latin) "cheerful." Hil-

lary Rodham Clinton, First Lady of the U.S.
Also: **Hillarey, Hillary.**

Hilda: (Teutonic) "battle maiden."
Also: **Heidi, Hilde, Hildie, Hildy.**

Hildegard: (Teutonic) "battle maiden." Hildegarde Howard, 19th-century paleontologist.
Also: **Hildagard, Hildagarde, Hilde; plus all diminutives of Hilda.**

Hilla: Hilla Rebay, museum director.

Hina: (HEE-nah) (Hawaiian) Mythology: Hawaiian goddess of the fishes.

Holland: (Dutch) "woodland"; place name.

Hollis: variant of Holly. Hollis Stacy, golfer.
Also: **Hollice.**

Holly: (Anglo-Saxon) "the holly tree." Holly Golightly, of Truman Capote's *Breakfast at Tiffany's* (1958).
Also: **Hollie, Hollin, Hollis.**

Honey: (Anglo-Saxon) "sweet one."

Honora: (Latin) "honorable." Honor Blackman, actress.
Also: **Honor, Honore (Fr), Honoria, Nora.**

Hope: (Anglo-Saxon) "hope; optimism."

Horatia: (Latin) "keeper of the hours." Feminine form of Horace.

Hortense, Hortensia: (Latin) "gardener." Hortense Calisher, writer; Hortensia Ma-

ria Alvirez, Mexican-American entrepreneur.
Also: **Hortencia, Hortensa.**

Hua: (Hwa) (Chinese) "magnificent; blossom." Hua Mulan, famed woman warrior of China (A.D. 400). Traditionally combined with another name.

Huberta: (Old German) feminine of Hubert.

Huette: (Old English) feminine of Hugh.
Also: **Hughette.**

Hulda: (Old German) "gracious or beloved."

Hunter: (Old English) "the hunter." Hunter Reno, model.

Hyacinth: (Greek) the flower or purple color.
Also: **Hyacintha, Jacinthe.** See also Jacinda.

Hyatt: (Old English) "from the high gate."
Also: **Hiatt.**

Hypatia: (Greek) "highest." Hypatia, 5th-century philosopher and mathematician.

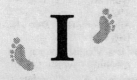

Ianthe: (Greek) a purple-colored flower.
Also: **Ian, Iolanthe.**

Ibernia: (Celtic) ancient name of Ireland.

Ida: (Teutonic) "happy." Ida Tarbell, journalist.
Also: **Idalla, Idella, Idelle.**

Idamae: (Greek/Anglo-Saxon) "happy kinswoman."

Idelia: (Teutonic) "noble."

Idelle: see Ida.

Iduna: (Old Norse) "lover."

Ignacia: (Latin) "fiery, ardent one."
Also: **Ignatia.**

Igraine: in Arthurian legend, the mother of Arthur.
Also: **Igrayne.**

Ila: (Old French) "from the island."

Ilana: (Hebrew) "tree."

Ileana: (Greek) "pertaining to ancient Illium or Troy." Ileana Ros-Lehtinen, first Hispanic woman elected to the U.S. Congress.
Also: **Ilea.**

Ilenna: (Greek) "from the city of Ilion or Troy."

Ilene, Iline, Illene, Illona: see Aileen.

Ilima: (Hawaiian) a Hawaiian flowering shrub.

Ilka: (Celtic) "hard worker."
Also: **Ilke.**

Ilona: (Hungarian) "beautiful one."

Ilsa, Ilse: variant of Elsa. Also see Elizabeth.

Iluminada: (Spanish) "illuminated."
Also: **Lumina.**

Imani: (Swahili) "faith." Iman, model.
Also: **Iman, Imaan.**

Imelda: (Italian) "fighter."

Imogene: (Latin) "an image." Imogen Cunningham, photographer.
Also: **Emagene, Emogene.**

Imperia: (Latin) "imperial one."

Ina: *see* Katherine.

India: (English) the name of the country.

Indira: (Sanskrit) "splendid." Indira Gandhi, former prime minister of India.

Indra: the Hindu god of rain and thunder.

Inez: (Spanish) "chaste; pure; gentle."
Also: **Ines.**

Inga: *see* Ingrid.

Ingrid: (Swedish) "Hero's daughter." The Norse goddess of fertility. Ingrid Bergman, actress.
Also: **Inga, Inge, Ingeborg.**

Iniga: (Latin) "fiery, ardent one."

Iola: (Greek) "dawn cloud; violet color."

Iolanthe: (Greek) "violet flower."
Also: **Ianthe.**

Iona: (Latin) The Hebridean island of Iona, an ancient religious site, was settled in 563 by St. Columba, who founded its monastery. This formed a base for the spread of Christianity through Scotland and northern England. Ione Skye, actress.
Also: **Ione, Ionia.**

Iphigenia: (Greek) "sacrifice."

Mythology: the daughter of Agamemnon. Iphigene Ochs Sulzberger, publisher.

Irene: (Greek) "peace." Irene of Athens, Byzantine empress.
Also: **Eirene, Irena, Irina, Rena, Rene, Reni, Rennie, Renny.**

Iris: (Greek) "rainbow." Iris, Greek goddess of the rainbow, inspired Juno to commemorate her forever with a flower that would bear Iris' name and bloom in the rainbow colors of Iris' robes.
Also: **Irisa, Irisha.**

Irma: (Teutonic) "strong."
Also: **Erma, Erme, Irme, Irmina, Irmine.**

Isa: (Old German) "iron-willed one."

Isabel: (Hebrew/Spanish) "consecrated to God." Originally from the name Elizabeth. Isabella I, queen of Castile; Isabel Allende, Chilean novelist.
Also: **Bel, Bella, Belle, Isabella, Isabelle, Isbel, Isobel, Isobella, Ysabel.**

Isadora: (Greek) "a gift." Feminine of Isidore. Isadora Duncan, dancer (1877–1927).
Also: **Dora, Dori, Dory, Isidora, Issy, Izzy.**

Isla: a Scottish river name meaning "swiftly flowing."

Isolde: (Celtic) "the fair." The lover of Tristan in Celtic legend.
Also: **Isolda.**

Ita: (Old Irish Gaelic) "thirst." St. Ita, a popular Irish saint.

Ivah: (Hebrew) "God's gracious gift."
Also: **Iva.**

Ivana: (Czech) feminine form of Ivan.
Also: **Ivania, Ivanka, Ivanna.**

Ivelisse: combination of Yvette and Lisa.
Also: **Yvelisse.**

Ivette: variant of Yvette.

Ivonne: variant of Yvonne.

Ivory: (Latin) "made of ivory."

Ivy: (English) an evergreen vine. Ivie Anderson, jazz vocalist (1905–1949); Ivy Baker Priest, treasurer of the U.S.
Also: **Iva, Ivey, Ivie.**

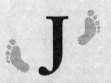

Jacinda/Jacinta: (Greek) "beautiful; hyacinth flower."
Also: **Giacinta, Jacenta, Jacinthe.** See also Hyacinth.

Jackie: (English) a short form of Jacqueline.

Jacoba: (Hebrew) "the supplanter." Feminine of Jacob.
Also: **Jackie, Jacobine.**

Jacqueline: (Hebrew) "the supplanter." Feminine of Jacques. Jacqueline Bouvier Kennedy Onassis, First Lady of the U.S., editor; Jacque Mercer, Miss America.
Also: **Jacki, Jackie, Jacklin, Jacklyn, Jackqueline, Jacky,**
Jaclin, Jaclyn, Jacquelin, Jacquelyn, Jacquenetta, Jacquenette, Jacquetta, Jacquette, Jacqui, Jaquelin, Jaquelyn, Jaquenetta, Jaquenette.

Jada: (Hebrew) "wise"; the jade stone. Jada Pinkett, actress.
Also: **Jadah, Jadda.**

Jade: (Spanish) "jade stone."

Jael: (Hebrew) "Jah is God." Jael Mbogo, Kenyan politician.

Jahia: (Arabic/Swahili) "prominent."
Also: **Jaha.**

Jaime: see Jamie.

Jama: (Sanskrit) "daughter."

Jamaica: the name of the Caribbean island. Jamaica Kincaid, author.

Jamie: a feminine form of James.
Also: **Jaime, Jaymee.**

Jamilla: (Arabic) "beautiful."
Also: **Djamila, Jamila.**

Jan: see Jane.

Jana: (YAH-nah) (Polish) feminine of Jan.
Also: **Janah, Janalyn, Janna, Jannah.**

Jane: (Hebrew) "God's gracious gift." Feminine of John. Jane Alexander, actress, chairwoman of the National Endowment for the Arts; Jane Goodall, primatologist.
Also: **Gian, Gianna, Giovanna (It), Jain, Jan, Janelle, Janet, Janette, Janey, Janice, Janie, Janna, Jayne, Jean, Jeanette,**

Jeanie, Jeanne (Fr), Jeannine, Joan, Joana, Joanie, Joanna, Johanna, Jone, Jonie, Juana, Juanita (Sp), Seana, Sheena, Sinead.

Janet, Janette, Janice: *see* Jane.

Janice: variant of Jane. Janis Joplin, rock singer.

Janna: an abbreviated form of Johanna.
Also: **Jana.**

Jardine: (French) "dweller near the garden."
Also: **Jardin.**

Jarita: (Hindustani) in East Indian legend, a bird mother who protected her four sons in a burning forest, whereupon her race became human.

Jarvia: feminine of Jarvis.

Jasmine, Jassamyn: (Persian) "fragrant flower." Jessamyn West, author.
Also: **Jasmin, Jasmina, Jazmin, Jessamine, Yasmine.**

Jasper: (Persian) "treasure bringer." The English name of one of the three Magi; also a semiprecious stone.

Jay: (Latin) the jaybird. Also used as a short form of names beginning with J-.
Also: **Jaye.**

Jaya: (Sanskrit) "victorious."

Jayne: (Sanskrit) "victorious one."

Jean, Jeanette, Jeanne: *see* Jane. Jeane Kirkpatrick, U.N. ambassador; Jeana Yeager, first woman to fly nonstop around the world without refueling (1986).

Jeannine: a form of Jane.
Also: **Janine, Jenyne.**

Jemima: (Hebrew) "dove."
Also: **Jemimah, Jemma, Jemmima, Mima.**

Jemma: *see* Gemma.

Jenna: (Arabic) "a small bird."
Also: **Jena.**

Jennifer, Jenny: (Welsh) "white; fair." A form of Guinevere.
Also: **Gennifer, Jenifer, Jenn, Jenna, Jenny.**

Jenny: *see* Jennifer.

Jeraldine: *see* Geraldine.

Jeremia: (Hebrew) "exalted of the Lord."
Also: **Jeremy, Jerri, Jerry.**

Jericho: (Hebrew) "his moon or month"; the biblical place name.

Jerri, Jerrie, Jerry: *see* Geraldine, Jeremia. Jerry Hall, model.

Jesse: a form of Jessica. Jessie Field, founder of the 4-H Club (1901). *See also* Jasmine.

Jesseline: (Hebrew) "wealthy woman."
Also: **Jesslyn.**

Jessica: (Hebrew) "rich; grace of God." Jessica Tandy, actress; Jessye Norman, opera singer. Feminine of Jesse.
Also: **Jess, Jessamine, Jesse, Jessi, Jessie, Jessy.**

Jetta: from jet, a black gemstone.

Jewel: (Latin) "a precious stone."
Also: **Jewell, Jewelyn.**

Jian: (Chinese) "strong." Traditionally combined with a second name.

Jill: *see* Julia.

Jillian: (Latin) "young, downy-haired child."
Also: **Gillian, Jill, Julia.**

Jinny: *see* Virginia.

Jiselle: variant of Giselle.

Jo: a short form of Joanna, Josephine, and other names beginning Jo-. Jo March, *Little Women* heroine (1868).

Joan: (Latin) feminine of John and a form of Jane. St. Joan of Arc.
Also: **Joni.**

Joanna, Joanne: forms of Jane.
Also: **Jo, Joana, Joann, Jo Ann, Johanna.**

Joaquina: (Spanish) feminine form of Joaquin.

Jobina: (Hebrew) "the afflicted."
Also: **Jobie, Jobyna.**

Jocelyn: (Latin) "fair; just."
Also: **Jocelin, Joscelin, Joslyn, Joycelin, Lyn, Lynn.**

Jocosa: (Latin) "humorous."

Jodie, Jody: forms of Judith. Jodie Foster, actress, director.

Joelle: (Hebrew) "Jehovah is God." Feminine of Joel.
Also: **Joell, Joella.**

Joely: *see* Joelle. Joely Fisher, actress.

Johanna: *see* Joanna.

Joi: *see* Joy. Joie Lee, actress.

Joice: *see* Joyce.

Jolan: (YOH-lawn) (Hungarian) variant of Yolanda; a flower name.

Jolanta: (Polish) "violet blossoms."

Jolene: a combination of Jo and Lena; variant of Jolie.
Also: **Jolean, Joleen, Jolena, Jolyn.**

Jolie: (French) "pretty."
Also: **Jolene.**

Joni: a form of Joan. Joni Mitchell, singer, songwriter.

Jonquil: a flower name.

Jordan: (Hebrew) "flowing down." Biblical: the river where Jesus was baptized.
Also: **Giordana, Jordain, Jordana (Sp), Jourdan, Jourdana.**

Josefina: (Hoh-seh-FEE-nah) *see* Josephine.

Josephine: (Hebrew) "she shall add." Feminine of Joseph. Josephine, empress of France; Josefina Lopez, playwright.
Also: **Fifi, Fina, Jo, Joey, Josefina (Sp), Josepha, Josephina, Josette, Josey, Josie.**

Josie: a short form of Josephine.

Jovita: (Latin) "joyful."
Also: **Jovina.**

Joy: (Latin) "joyful."
Also: **Joi, Joie.**

Joyce: variant of Joy. Joyce Carol Oates, author.
Also: **Joice, Joy.**

Juanita: (Hebrew) "God is beneficent." Feminine of Juan.

Juanita Kreps, secretary of commerce.
Also: **Anita, Juana.**

Judith: (Hebrew) "admired; praised." Biblical: Book of Judith.
Also: **Jodie, Jody, Jude, Judi, Juditha, Judy, Judyta (Pol).**

Judson: the surname used as a first name. Judsen Culbreth, publishing executive.

Judy: see Judith.

Julia, Julian: (Greek) "youthful." Feminine of Julius. Julian of Norwich, British mystic and first English woman of letters (14th century).
Also: **Giuliana (It), Jill, Jule, Juli, Juliana, Juliane, Julie, Juliet, Julietta, Juliette.**

Julie: see Julia.

Juliet: see Julia. Shakespeare's heroine. Juliette Lewis, actress.

Jun: (Chinese) "truth." (Japanese) "obedient."

June: (Latin) the month.
Also: **Juneth, Junette, Junia, Junie.**

Junia: variant of June.

Juniata: the Juniata River in Pennsylvania. Came into use as a first name due to a popular 19th-century song.

Juno: (Latin) in Roman mythology, the queen of the heavens and goddess of marriage and maternity. Her Greek counterpart is Hera.

Justice: a Puritan virtue name.

Justine: (Latin) "the just." Feminine of Justin.

Also: **Justina, Justyna (Pol), Tina.**

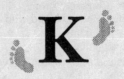

K

Kachina: (American Indian) "sacred dancer."
Also: **Kachine.**

Kai: (kye) (Hawaiian) "the sea."

Kaitlin: see Caitlin.
Also: **Kaitlyn, Katlin.**

Kala: (KAH-lah) "black; one of the names of the Hindu god Siva."

Kalama: (American Indian) "the wild goose."

Kalani: (Hawaiian) an invented name.

Kaldora: (Greek) "beautiful gift."

Kali: (KAH-lee) (Sanskrit) "energy." Wife of Shiva and the Hindu goddess of both creation and destruction.

Kalila: (kah-LEE-lah) (Arabic) "much loved."
Also: **Kalilah, Kylila.**

Kalina: (Polish) a flower and place name.

Kalma: (Teutonic) "calm."

Kama: (KAH-mah) (Sanskrit) "love." Mythology: the Hindu god of love.

Kamaria: (African) "moonlike."
Also: **Kamra.**

Kami: the Shinto divine powers associated with ancestors. Kami Cotler, actress.

Kamila, Kamilla: see Camilla. Also: **Kamilah.**

Karen, Karin, Karyn: see Katherine.

Karima: (Arabic/Swahili) "generous."

Karla: see Carla.

Karma: (Sanskrit) "destiny." Also: **Carma.**

Karmel: variant of Carmela.

Karol: see Carol.

Karolina, Karoline, Karolyn: see Caroline.

Kasey: a form of Casey.

Kasmira: (Old Slavic) "commands peace."

Kassandra: a form of Cassandra.

Kassie: variant of Cassie and short form of names beginning Kas-.

Kat: see Katherine.

Kate: see Katherine.

Kateri: a form of Katherine. Kateri Tekakwitha, the first North American Indian proposed for canonization by the Roman Catholic Church.

Kathe: see Katherine. Käthe Kollwitz, German artist.

Katherine: (Greek) "pure." Also: **Catherina, Catherine, Cathleen, Catrin (Welsh), Ekaterina, Kara, Karen, Karena, Karin, Karyn, Kat, Katarzyna (Pol), Kate, Katharina, Kathe, Kathleen, Kathlene, Kathryn, Katrina, Katrine, Kathie, Kathy,** **Katie, Ketti, Kit, Kittie, Kitty, Trina.**

Kathleen, Kathlene: see Katherine.

Kathy: see Katherine.

Katrina: see Katherine.

Kay: a short form of names beginning with K. Also given as an independent name. Mary Kay Ash, founder, Mary Kay Cosmetics; Kaye Lani Rae Rafko, Miss America. Also: **Cai (Welsh), Kayla.**

Kayla: a form of Kay. Also: **Cayla, Kaila.**

Kayleigh: a contemporary name. Also: **Kalie, Kayley.**

Kazu: (KAH-zoo) (Japanese) "peace." Also: **Kaz, Kazuko.**

Kearny: (Irish) "warlike; victorious."

Keely: (Irish Gaelic) "beautiful one." Keely Smith, singer. Also: **Keeley, Keelie.**

Keiki: (KAY-kee) (Hawaiian) "child." Also: **Keikilani.**

Keiko: (KAY-koh) (Japanese) "blessed child; joyous child." Also: **Kei.**

Keira: (Irish Gaelic) "little dark one." Also: **Kerr, Kiera, Kieren, Kieron.**

Keisha: (KEE-shah) see Keshia.

Kelda: (Old Norse) "a spring."

Kell: see Kelda.

Kelly: (Irish Gaelic) "warrior"; an Irish surname. Kellye Cash, Miss America.
Also: **Kellie.**

Kelsey: (Teutonic) "from the water."
Also: **Kelcey, Kelcie, Kelsie.**

Kendall: (Celtic) "valley of the River Kent."
Also: **Kendell.**

Kendra: a contemporary name; a combination of Ken and Sandra, Alexandra, or Andrea.
Also: **Kenna.**

Kenley: (Old English) "of the king's meadow."
Also: **Kenleigh.**

Kennedy: (Celtic) "chief of the clan"; Irish surname. Kennedy, TV personality.

Kenya: (African) "artist."

Kenyon: (Cornish) "fair-haired."

Kerensa: (Cornish) "affection, love."
Also: **Karenza, Kerenza.**

Kerrigan: an Irish surname.

Kerry: (Irish Gaelic) "dark one"; an Irish county name.
Also: **Keri, Kerrie.**

Keshia: (Hebrew) the shrub cassia. The name of one of Job's three beautiful daughters.
Also: **Kasia, Kezia, Keziah, Kizzie.**

Ketti: see Katherine.

Ketura: (Hebrew) "incense." Biblical: the second wife of Abraham.
Also: **Keturah.**

Kevina: (Celtic) "gentle."
Also: **Kevia.**

Kezia, Keziah: see Keshia.

Kiana: a contemporary name.
Also: **Keanna.**

Kiera: (Irish Gaelic) "little dark one."
Also: **Keira, Kerr, Kerry, Kieron.**

Kilie: see Kylie.

Kim: (Vietnamese) "gold."

Kimba: see Kimberly.

Kimberly: (Old English) "from the royal fortress meadow."
Also: **Kim, Kimba, Kimberlea, Kimberlee, Kimberley, Kimmy, Kym.**

Kimiko: (KEE-mee-koh) (Japanese) "righteous child." Kimiko Date, tennis player.
Also: **Kimi.**

Kineta: (Greek) "active one."

Kinu: (KEE-noo) (Japanese) silk.

Kiona: (American Indian) "brown hills."

Kirby: (Anglo-Saxon) "from the church town."
Also: **Kirbee, Kirbie.**

Kiri: (Maori) "bell." Kiri Te Kanawa, soprano.

Kirsten: Scandinavian form of Christine.
Also: **Kiersten, Kirstin, Kirsty.** See also Kristen.

Kit, Kitty: a form of Katherine. Kitty Carlisle Hart.

Klarissa: see Clarissa.

Kleantha: (Greek) a flower name.

Klymene: (Greek) "celebrated."

Kora: (Greek) "maiden."
Also: **Kore, Koren.** *See also*
Cora.

Koren: *see* Kora.

Krista: Czech form of Christine.
Also: **Krysta.**

Kristen, Kristin: (Scandinavian) a form of Christine,
Kristi Yamaguchi, skater.
Also: **Kirsten, Krista, Kristan,
Kristine, Kristy, Krystian.**

Krystal: a form of Crystal.
Also: **Kristal, Krystle.**

Kyla: (Gaelic) "comely."

Kyle: (Gaelic) "a narrow
piece of land"; a Scottish
district.

Kylie: a popular contemporary
name.
Also: **Kilie.**

Kyna: (Irish Gaelic) "intelligence, wisdom."

Kyra: (Greek) "lord." Kyra
Sedgwick, actress.

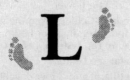

Lacey: French place name
used as a surname or first
name.
Also: **Lacie, Lacy.**

Laila: *see* Leila.

Laine: *see* Elaine.

Lake: the English word used
as a first name. Also a surname meaning "dweller by
the brook or stream."

Lala: (Slavic) the tulip.

Lalita: (Sanskrit) "pleasing."

Lana: *see* Alana.

Lane: (Middle English) "from
the narrow road." Lane Bryant, entrepreneur.
Also: **Laina, Laine, Lanette,
Laney, Lanie, Lanny, Layne.**

Lani: (LAH-nee) (Hawaiian)
"sky; heaven; royal child."

Lantana: a flowering shrub.

Lara: (Latin) "well-known."

Laraine: *see* Lorraine.

Larissa: (Greek) "cheerful
one." Larissa Latynina, Russian gymnast.
Also: **Larisa, Laryssa.**

Lark: (Middle English) the
songbird celebrated for its
beautiful song during flight.
Lark Song Previn, child of
actress Mia Farrow and conductor Andre Previn.

Latonia, LaToya: (Greek) Latona, the Roman deity and
mother of Apollo and Diana. LaToya Jackson, singer.
Also: **Latona, Latonya, Tonya.**

Laura: (Latin) "the laurel."
Feminine of Lawrence.
Also: **Lari, Laureen, Laurel,
Lauren, Laurette, Lora, Loralie,
Loree, Lorelie, Loren, Loretta,
Lorette, Lori, Lorie, Lorinda,
Lorine, Lorna, Lorne, Lorrie.**

Laurel: the laurel tree, symbol
of victory.

Lauren: a form of Laura.
Also: **Laurin, Loren.**

Laurette: *see* Laura. Lauretta
Freeman, basketball player.

Laveda: (Latin) "purified one."

Laverne: (French) "from the grove of alder trees."
Also: **Laverna, LaVerne, Vern, Verna, Verne.**

Lavinia: (Latin) "woman of Rome; purified." Mythology: the second wife of Aeneas, the Trojan hero.
Also: **Lavina, Vina, Vinia.**

Layla: see Leila.

Leah: (Hebrew) "the weary." Biblical: the wife of Jacob.
Also: **Lea, Leda, Leigh, Lia (It), Lida.**

Leandra: (Latin) "lioness." Feminine of Leander.

Leanne: combination of Lee and Anne.
Also: **Liana, Lianne.**

Leatrice: combination of Leah and Beatrice.

Leda: see Alida, Leah. Mythology: the mother of Helen of Troy.

Lee: (Anglo-Saxon) "meadow." (Chinese) "plum." Lee Krasner, artist.
Also: **Lea, Leigh.**

Leigh: see Lee.

Leila: (Arabic) "black; dark as night."
Also: **Laila, Layla, Leela, Leilah, Lila, Lilah.**

Leilani: (lay-LAH-nee) (Hawaiian) "heavenly flower." Leilani Estavan, basketball player, student.

Lela, Lelah, Lelia: see Lillian.

Lemuela: (Hebrew) "con-

secrated to God." Feminine of Lemuel.

Lena, Lina: a diminutive of Helena and Carolina, also used as an independent name. Lena Horne, singer.

Lenore, Leonora, Leonore: see Helen.

Leola: a feminine form of Leo. See also Leona.

Leoma: (Old English) "light, brightness."

Leona: (Latin) "the lion." Another feminine form of Leo. Leonie Adams, poet.
Also: **Lee, Lennie, Lenny, Leola, Leone, Leoni, Leonie.**

Leonarda: (Old Frankish) "lion-brave."

Leontine: (Latin) "brave as a lion." Another form of Leo. Leontyne Price, opera singer.

Leopoldine: (Old German) "bold for the people."

Leotie: (American Indian) "prairie flower."

Lesley: (Celtic) "from the gray fort." Feminine of Leslie.
Also: **Les, Lesleigh, Leslie, Lesly.**

Leta: see Letitia.

Letitia: (Latin) "joy; delight." Letitia Baldrige, authority on etiquette.
Also: **Laetitia, Leta, Leticia, Letizia, Lettie, Letty, Tish.**

Lettie, Letty: see Charlotte, Letitia.

Levana: (Latin) the Roman goddess, protector of children.

Lewanna: (Hebrew) "the

beaming white one; the moon."

Li Chen: (Chinese) "beautiful treasure."

Lia: see Leah.

Lian: (LEE-ahn) (Chinese) "willow tree."
Also: **Liane, Lianne.**

Liana: (French) a name from nature; the liana vine.
Also: **Lianna.**

Libby: see Elizabeth.

Liberty: a contemporary name.

Lida: (Slavonic) "loved by all."
Also: **Lyda, Lilah, Lilla.** See also Alida, Delilah, Leah. Lila, Lillian.

Lidia: see Lydia.

Lien Hua: (Chinese) "lotus flower."

Liesl: German form of Elizabeth.
Also: **Liezl, Lisl.**

Liki: (LEE-kee) (Hawaiian) "rainbow."

Lila: (Persian) lilac.
Also: **Lilac.**

Lilabel: (Persian) "beautiful lily."

Lilac: (Persian) a bluish color; a lilac flower.

Lilith: (East Semitic) "belonging to the night." According to folklore, Lilith was the first wife of Adam. She was expelled from Eden and replaced by Eve.
Also: **Lilly, Lily.**

Lilka: (Polish) "famous warrior maiden."

Lillian: (Latin) "a lily." Lillian Hellman, playwright.
Also: **Lela, Lelah, Lelia, Lil, Lila, Lilah, Lilia, Lilian, Lilla, Lilli, Lillie, Lilly, Lily, Lilyan.**

Lillie, Lilly, Lily: see Lillian.

Lillith: see Lilith.

Lilybelle: (Latin) "the beautiful lily."
Also: **Lillibel, Lilybell, plus all forms of Lillian.**

Lin: (Chinese) "jade."

Lina: a short form of names ending -leen, -lena, -lene, -lina, and -line.

Linda: (Spanish) "beautiful." Also a diminutive of Belinda. Linda Ronstadt, pop singer.
Also: **Lind, Lindie, Lindy, Lynd, Lynda.**

Lindsay, Lindsey: (Old English) "from the linden tree island." Lindsay Crouse, actress.
Also: **Linsey, Lynsey.**

Linnea: (Old Norse) lime tree.

Linnet: the linnet bird.
Also: **Linet, Linette, Lynette, Lynnette.**

Liora: (Israeli) "light."

Lisa, Lise, Lissa, Liz, Liza, Lizzie, Lizzy: forms of Elizabeth. Lise Meitner, Austrian scientist who pioneered splitting of the atom but refused to participate in creating the atom bomb (1878–1968).
Also: **Leesa.**

Lisabet, Lisabeth, Lisbeth: see Elizabeth.

Lisl: see Liesl.

Liva: *see* Olivia.

Liz: a familiar form of Elizabeth. Liz Smith, columnist.

Liza: a familiar form of Elizabeth. Liza Minnelli, singer.

Loie: *see* Louise. Loie Fuller, founder of free expression in dance (1862–1928).

Lois: (Greek) "battle maiden." A feminine form of Louis. *See also* Aloysia, Louise.

Lola: (Spanish) "strong woman." A feminine form of Charles.
Also: **Loleta, Lolita.** *See also* Theola.

Lolita: a Spanish form of Lola. Lolita Davidovich, actress.

Lora: *see* Laura.

Loraine, Lorainne: *see* Lorraine.

Lorelei: (Teutonic) "alluring." Mythology: sirens of the Rhine River.
Also: **Loralei, Loralie.**

Loren: *see* Lauren.

Lorena: variant of Laura, Lorraine.

Loretta: *see* Laura. Loretta Lynn, country singer.

Lori, Lorie, Lorrie: *see* Laura.

Lorine: *see* Laura.

Lorna: *see* Laura.

Lorraine: (Teutonic) "famous in battle."
Also: **Laraine, Loraine, Lorena.**

Lotta, Lotte, Lottie, Lotty: *see* Charlotte.

Lotus: (Egyptian) "flower of the lotus tree; bloom of forgetfulness."

Louanne: (Teutonic) "gracious war heroine."

Louella: *see* Luella.

Louise: (Teutonic) "battle maiden." Another feminine form of Louis. Louisa May Alcott, *Little Women* author.
Also: **Aloysia, Eloise, Heloise, Lou, Louella, Louisa, Lova, Lovisa, Loyce, Luisa (It, Sp).**

Lourdes: a town in southwestern France, site of religious visions by St. Bernadette. Lourdes G. Baird, California state attorney general, judge.

Lova: a form of Lovisa or Louise.

Love: the English word used as a surname and first name.

Lovisa: a form of Louise.

Luana: (Old German-Hebrew) "graceful battle maid."

Luba: (Slavonic) "lover."
Also: **Lubba.**

Lucia: a form of Lucy.

Lucille: *see* Lucy. Lucille Ball, comedienne.

Lucinda: a form of Lucy.

Lucretia: meaning unclear; could be considered a form of Lucy. Lucretia Mott, antislavery activist (1793–1880).
Also: **Lucrecia, Lucrezia.**

Lucy: (Latin) "light." Feminine of Lucius. Lucy Stone, the first American woman to keep her own name after marriage (1818–1893).
Also: **Lu, Lucia, Lucie, Lucilla, Lucille, Lucinda, Lucretia, Lulu.**

Ludella: (Old English) "famous elf."

Ludmilla: (Old Slavic) "beloved by the people."
Also: **Ludmila.**

Luella: (Latin) "the appeaser." Louella Parsons, gossip columnist.
Also: **Lou, Louella, Lu.**

Lulu: (Arabic) *see* Lucy. "pearl."

Lumina: (Latin) "illuminates."
Also: **Luminosa.** *See also* Iluminada.

Luna: (Latin) "moon." Roman goddess of the moon.
Also: **Lunette.**

Lupe: *see* Guadalupe.

Lydia: (Greek) "woman of Lydia."
Also: **Liddy, Lidia, Lydie.**

Lynda: variant of Linda.

Lynette: *see* Linnet.

Lynn: (Old English) "waterfall." Also a form of Evelyn, Madeline.
Also: **Lyn, Lynna, Lynne.**

Lynsey: *see* Lindsay.

Lyris: (Greek) "of the music of the lyre; lyrical."
Also: **Liris, Lyric.**

Lysandra: (Greek) "liberator of men." Feminine of Lysander.

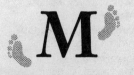

Mabel: (Latin) "lovable." Mabel Mercer, cabaret singer.
Also: **Belle, Mable, Mae.** *See also* Maybelle.

Mackenzie: (Scottish) "son of Kenzie."

Madalon, Madelon: forms of Madeleine.

Maddie, Maddy: short forms of Madeleine and other names beginning Mad-.

Madeleine: (English/French) "woman of Magdala." Madeleine Albright, U.N. ambassador.
Also: **Mada, Madalon, Madalyn, Maddie, Madelaine, Madelene, Madeline, Madelon, Madlen, Magda, Magdalen, Magdalena (Sp), Marleen, Marlene, Marline.**

Madge: *see* Margaret.

Madhur: (Hindi) "sweet."

Madison: (Teutonic) "mighty in battle."
Also: **Maddie, Maddy.**

Madlen: *see* Madeleine.

Madonna: (Latin) "my lady." Madonna, pop singer.
Also: **Madona.**

Madora: (Greek) "a gift."

Madra: (Latin) "mother."
Also: **Madre.**

Mae: *see* May.

Maeve: (Irish) "joy." In Irish legend, the queen of the province Connaught. Maeve Binchy, author.

Magda, Magdalen: *see* Madeleine.

Magena: (American Indian) "the coming moon."

Maggie: short form of Margaret.
Also: **Maggy.**

Magnolia: (Anglo-Saxon) the magnolia tree. Magnolia Hawks, of Edna Ferber's *Show Boat* (1926).

Mahala: (American Indian) "woman."

Mahalia: (Hebrew) "tenderness." Mahalia Jackson, singer.
Also: **Mahala, Mehalia.**

Mahina: (mah-HEE-nah) (Hawaiian) "moon; moonlight."

Mahita: (Sanskrit) "celebrated."

Mai, Maia: (French) "May." Maia, Roman goddess of spring. Mai Zetterling, Swedish film director. *See also* May, Maya.

Maida: (Anglo-Saxon) "maiden."
Also: **Maddie, Maidy, Mayda.**

Maile: (Hawaiian) a native Hawaiian shrub, a type of periwinkle.

Mairead: Mairead Corrigan, cofounder of Ulster Peace Movement, youngest winner of Nobel Peace Prize (b. 1944).

Maisie: *see* Margaret.

Majesta: (Latin) "majestic one."

Makana: (Hawaiian) "gift."

Malia: (Hawaiian) variant of Mary.

Malika: (Swahili/Arabic) "queen."

Maliko: (Hawaiian) "to bud."

Malina: (Hawaiian) "calming, soothing."

Mallory: (Latin) "luckless."

Malva: (Greek) "soft, slender"; a flower name.

Malvina: (origin uncertain) Malvina Hoffman, sculptor.

Mamie: *see* Mary. Mamie Eisenhower, First Lady of the U.S.

Mana: (MAH-nuh) (Hawaiian) "supernatural powers."

Mandy: a familiar form of Amanda.

Manon: *see* Mary. Manon Roland, French Revolution heroine.

Mansi: (Hopi Indian) "plucked flower."

Manuela: (Spanish) "God is with us." Manuela Saenz, Ecuadoran revolutionary, wife of Simón Bolívar.

Mara: *see* Damara, Mary, Samara.

Marceline: (Latin) "of Mars; warlike"; a semiprecious rose-pink stone.
Also: **Marcelina, Marcelite.**

Marcella: *see* Marceline, Marcia.
Also: **Marcela.**

Marcia: (Latin) "of Mars; warlike." Feminine of Mark.
Also: **Marceline, Marcella, Marcie, Marcy, Markita, Marsha.**

Mare: *see* Mary. Mare Winningham, actress.

Margaret: (Greek) "a pearl." Margaret I, queen of Denmark, Norway, Sweden; Margaret Mead, anthropologist.
Also: **Gredel, Greta, Gretchen**

(Ger), Madge, Mag, Maggie, Maisie, Margarita (Sp), Marge, Margery, Margie, Margita, Margo, Margot, Margrethe, Marguerita, Marguerite, Marjorie, Meg, Peg, Peggy.

Margery, Marjorie: *see* Margaret.

Margita: (MAHR-gee-tah) variant of Margaret.

Margo: *see* Margaret. Margo Jones, theatrical producer. Also: **Margaux, Margeaux, Margot.**

Margrethe: a form of Margaret. Margrethe II, queen of Denmark.

Marguerite: French form of Margaret. Marguerite Duras, writer, filmmaker.

Mari: a form of Mary. Mari Evans, writer.

Maria: a form of Mary. Maria Callas, opera singer; Maria Montessori, educator.

Mariah: a form of Mary. Mariah Carey, singer.

Marian, Marion: forms of Mary. Marianne Moore, poet.

Maribel: (Latin) a combination of Mary and Belle. Maribel Atienzar, bullfighter.

Marie: a French form of Mary.

Mariel: a form of Mary. Mariel Hemingway, actress.

Marietta, Mariette, Minette: *see* Mary. Marietta Tree, first woman U.S. ambassador to the United Nations.

Marigolde: (Anglo-Saxon) the marigold flower. The marigold was the symbol of the Virgin Mary. Also: **Marigold.**

Marika: a form of Mary.

Marilis: short form of Amaryllis.

Marilla: (Hebrew) "Mary of the fine mind." Marilla Ricker, first American woman to vote (1870).

Marilyn: a form of Mary. Also: **Marilynne, Marylin, Marylon.**

Marina: (Latin) "of the sea." Marina, Mexican Indian princess, mistress of Cortés. Also: **Marena, Marinna, Marnie.**

Mariposa: (Spanish) "butterfly"; a flower name.

Maris: (Latin) "sea star." Also: **Mari, Marisa, Marras, Marris, Merisa.**

Marisa: *see* Maris. Marisa Tomei, actress.

Marisol: (origin uncertain) Marisol, artist.

Maristan: (Latin) "in Mary's service."

Marjani: (Swahili) "coral."

Marjorie: a form of Margaret.

Mark, Marketa: Czech form of Margaret. Also: **Markie, Marquetta.**

Marla: *see* Mary. Also: **Marlo.**

Marleen, Marlene, Marline: *see* Madeline. Marlene Dietrich, actress.

Marlo: *see* Mary. Marlow Moss, artist.

Marmara: (Greek) "flashing, glittering."

Marni: a familiar form of Marina.
Also: **Marney, Marnie.**

Marquesa: (Latin) "to break." The Marquesas Islands are part of French Polynesia.

Marsha: see Marcia.

Marta: see Martha.

Martha: (Aramaic) "lady." Biblical: sister of Lazarus. Martha Graham, creator of modern dance; Martha Coolidge, film director.
Also: **Marta, Martella, Marthe (Fr, Ger), Marti, Martie, Matti, Mattie.**

Martika: Martika, Cuban-American singer.

Martina: (Latin) "belonging to Mars." Feminine of Martin. Martina Navratilova, tennis player.
Also: **Marta, Marteena, Marti, Martine, Teena, Tina.**

Marva: (Latin) "wonderful."
Also: **Marvel, Marvella.**

Marvel: see Marva.

Marvina: feminine of Marvin.

Mary: (Hebrew) "bitter." Biblical: the mother of Jesus. Mary, Queen of Scots.
Also: **Malia, Mamie, Manon, Mara, Mare, Mari, Maria, Mariah, Mariam, Marian, Marie, Mariel, Marietta, Mariette, Marilyn, Marion, Marla, Marlo, Marya, Maureen, Mimi, Minette, Miriam, Mitzi, Mitzie, Moira (Irish), Moll, Mollie, Molly, Morene, Polly.**

Maryann: a combination of Mary and Ann.
Also: **Marianne, Mary Ann, Mary Anne.**

Marybeth: a combination of Mary and Beth. Other combinations include Maryellen, Maryjo, and Marylou.

Mathea: (Hebrew) "God-given."
Also: **Mattia, Matty.**

Mathilda: (Teutonic) "brave in battle."
Also: **Matti, Matty, Maud, Maude, Tilda, Tillie, Tilly.**

Matima: (Swahili) "full moon."

Matsuko: (MAHT-soo-koh) (Japanese): pine tree.
Also: **Matsu.**

Maud, Maude: see Mathilda.

Maureen: see Mary.

Maurita: (Latin) "little dark girl."
Also: **Marita, Mauretta, Mauri, Rita.**

Mavis: (Celtic) the name of a songbird. Mavis Staples, singer.
Also: **Mavia.**

Maxine: (Latin) "greatest." Maxine Hong Kingston, novelist. Feminine of Maximillian.

May: (Latin) "Maia, the month of May."
Also: **Mae, Mai, Maya.**

Maya: (Spanish) variant of Maia. (Hindustani) "illusion." (Sanskrit) "art and wisdom of supernatural power." Maya Lin, architect; Maya Deren, experimental filmmaker.

Maybelle: a combination of

May and Belle. Mother Maybelle Carter, the "First Lady of Country Music."
Also: **Maybella.**

Mayda: (English) "maiden."
Also: **Maidie.**

Medea: (Greek) "part goddess; sorceress." Mythology: the enchantress who helped Jason, of the Argonauts, obtain the Golden Fleece.

Medina: (Arabic) "city of the prophet." Medina, the second-holiest city in Islam (after Mecca).

Meg: see Margaret.

Megan: (Celtic) "the strong."
Also: **Meagan, Meg, Meghan.**

Mehetabel: (Hebrew) "one of God's favored."
Also: **Mehitabel, Metabel.**

Mei Hua: (may-hooah) (Chinese) a plum blossom, the symbol of beauty and longevity.

Mei Li: (may-lee) (Chinese) "beautiful; enchanting."

Melanie: (Greek) "darkness; clad in black."
Also: **Lani, Lanny, Malan, Mel, Melan, Melania, Melina, Mellie, Melly.**

Melantha: (Greek) "dark flower."

Melba: see Melvina.

Melika: (Greek) "lyrical."

Melina: see Malina, Melanie.

Melissa: (Greek) "honeybee."
Also: **Mel, Melisa, Missy.**

Melita: "honey"; the Latin name for the island of Malta.
Also: **Melida.**

Melody: (Greek) "song."
Also: **Melodie.**

Melosa: (Spanish) "gentle."

Melrosa: (Latin) "honey of roses."

Melvina: Feminine of Melvin.
Also: **Malvina, Melba, Melva.**

Mena: see Philomena.

Meralda: short form of Esmeralda.

Mercedes: (Spanish) "merciful." Mercedes Ruehl, actress.
Also: **Merci, Mercy.**

Mercy: (English) "mercy." A Puritan virtue name. Mercy Otis Warren, 18th-century poet.
Also: **Mercia.**

Meredith: (Celtic) "protector of the sea." Meredith Monk, choreographer. Meredyth.

Meriel: see Muriel.

Merisa: see Maris.

Merle: (Latin) "blackbird." Meryl Streep, actress.
Also: **Merl, Merla, Merrill, Meryl.**

Merrie: (Anglo-Saxon) "joyous; merry."
Also: **Meri, Merry.**

Merritt: (Anglo-Saxon) "of merit."
Also: **Merri.**

Merry: see Merrie.

Mert, Merta: see Myrtle.

Mertice: (Old English) "famous; pleasant."

Meryl: see Merle.

Messina: (Latin) "a middle child."

Meta: (Latin) "ambitious." Meta Fuller, sculptor.

Metis: (Greek) "wisdom; skill."

Mia: (Latin) "mine." Mia Farrow, actress.

Miaou Miaou: (French) The sound a cat makes—as in meow meow. Miou-Miou, French actress.

Micah: a form of Michaela.

Michaela: (Hebrew) "Who is like God?" Feminine of Michael.
Also: **Michaeline, Michal, Michalin, Michelle, Mickie, Miguela, Mikaela, Mikayla.**

Michaeline: *see* Michaela.

Michelle: a form of Michaela.

Michiko: (MEE-chee-koh) (Japanese) "beautiful, wise child." Michiko, crown princess of Japan; Michiko Kakutani, book critic.
Also: **Michi.**

Midori: (mee-DOR-ee) (Japanese) "green." Midori Ito, skater.

Mignon: (French) "dainty." Mysterious girl in the popular opera *Mignon* (1866).
Also: **Mignot.**

Mika: (MEE-kah) (American Indian) "the raccoon."

Miki: (MEE-kee) (Japanese) "beautiful; stem."

Mila: (Czech) "loved by the people."
Also: **Milla.**

Milagros: (Spanish) "miracles."
Also: **Mila.**

Milcha: Milcha Sanchez-Scott, playwright.

Mildred: (Anglo-Saxon) "soft; gentle." Mildred Pierce, hardworking mother/entrepreneur of novel and film of the same name.
Also: **Mildrid, Milli, Millie.**

Miles: (Latin) "soldier." Miles Franklin, Australian writer.

Mililani: (Hawaiian) "beloved."

Millicent: (Teutonic) "strength." Melisande, queen of Jerusalem (c1105–1160).
Also: **Melicent, Melisande, Milicent, Milli, Millie, Milly, Missy.**

Millie, Milly: *see* Camilla, Emily, Mildred, Millicent.

Mimi: *see* Mary.

Mina: *see* Wilhelmina. (Hindi) "precious stone." Mina Stevens Fleming, astronomer (1857–1911).
Also: **Minette.**

Minda: (Hindi) "wisdom."

Minerva: (Greek) "wise." In Roman mythology, the goddess of wisdom, war, and arts and crafts.
Also: **Min, Minnie, Minny.**

Ming Yi: (Chinese) "brilliant and charming; joyful."

Minna: (Teutonic) "loving remembrance." A short form of Wilhelmina.
Also: **Mina, Minnie, Minny.**

Minnie, Minny: *see* Minerva.

Mir: (meer) (Czech) "peace."

Mira: (Latin) "wonderful one."
Also: **Mirella.** *See also* Almira, Mirabel, Miranda.

Mirabel: (Latin) "of great beauty."
Also: **Bell, Belle, Mira, Mirabelle.**

Miranda: (Latin) "to be admired." Miranda Richardson, actress.
Also: **Mandy, Mireille, Miri, Randie, Randy.**

Mireille: French form of Miranda.

Miriam: the original Hebrew form of Mary.

Mirth: (Teutonic) "merriment." *See also* Merrie.

Missy: a familiar form of Melissa, Millicent.

Misty: a contemporary name.

Mitzi: *see* Mary.

Modesta: (Latin) "shy; unassuming."
Also: **Desta, Deste, Modeste.**

Modesty: (Latin) "modest one."

Moira: an Irish form of Mary. Moira Shearer, ballerina.
Also: **Moyra.**

Mollie, Molly: forms of Mary.

Momilani: (Hawaiian) "pearl."
Also: **Momi.**

Momo: (Japanese) "peach."

Mona: (Latin) "the alone; the peaceful." *See also* Desdemona, Ramona.

Monet: contemporary name

inspired by Claude Monet, French Impressionist painter.

Monica: (Latin) "adviser." St. Monica; Monica Seles, tennis player.
Also: **Monique.**

Monserrat: (Latin) "jagged mountain." Montserrat Fontes, teacher, author.

Montana: (Latin) "mountain"; the Western state.

Monterey: (Spanish) "the king's forest." This California place name commemorates the county of Monterey, named after the viceroy of New Spain.

Moreen: *see* Mary.

Morela: (Polish) "apricot."

Morgan: (Old Welsh) "shore of the sea." Morgan Le Fay, sister of King Arthur.
Also: **Morgaine, Morgana, Morganne, Morgayne.**

Moriah: (Hebrew) a biblical place name.
Also: **Mariah.**

Morla: (Hebrew) "chosen by the Lord."

Morna: (Gaelic) "the tender and gentle."
Also: **Myrna.**

Moti: (Sanskrit) "pearl."
Also: **Motti.**

Mu Lan: (MOO-lahn) (Chinese) the magnolia blossom.

Muriel: (Celtic) "shining sea." Muriel Hazel Wright, American Indian activist.
Also: **Meriel, Murial, Murielle.**

Murphy: (Irish Gaelic) "sea

warrior." TV character Murphy Brown.

Myrna: (Gaelic) "beloved, gentle." Myrna Loy, actress.
Also: **Mirna, Moina.**

Myrtle: (Greek) a plant name.
Also: **Mert, Merta, Myrta.**

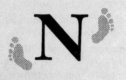

Nada: (Slavic) "hope."

Nadia: the Russian form of Hope. Nadja Salerno-Sonnenberg, violinist. Nadia Comaneci, Romanian gymnast.
Also: **Nadya.**

Nadine: (French) "hope." Nadine Gordimer, Nobel prize–winning author.
Also: **Nadene, Nadina.**

Nadiya: (Swahili) "generous."

Nafisa: (Swahili) "priceless."

Nairne: (Scotch Gaelic) "from the alder-tree river."

Nan: a form of Ann.

Nancy: a form of Ann.
Also: **Nance, Nancee, Nancey, Nanci, Nanette.**

Nanette: diminutive form of Ann. Nanette Fabray, actress.
Also: **Nanon.**

Naomi: (Hebrew) "sweet; pleasant." Biblical: the mother-in-law of Ruth. Naomi James, first woman to sail around the world;

Naomi Wolf, feminist, author.
Also: **Noemi (Sp), Nomi.**

Napea: (Latin) "she of the valleys."

Nara: (Japanese) "oak."

Narcissa: (Greek) "daffodil." Mythology: the beautiful youth who fell in love with his reflection in a pool and who was eventually transformed into the flower that bears his name.
Also: **Narcisse.**

Natalie: (Latin) "child of Christmas." A feminine form of Nathan. Natalia Makarova, ballerina.
Also: **Nat, Natala, Natale, Natalee, Natalia, Natasha, Nathalie, Natica, Natika, Nattie, Netta, Nettie, Netty, Talie.** See also Noel.

Natasha: see Natalie. Natasha Richardson, actress.

Nathania: (Hebrew) a feminine form of Nathan.

Natividad: (Spanish) "born at Christmas."

Neala: (Irish Gaelic) "champion." A feminine form of Neal.
Also: **Neely, Neila.**

Nebula: (Latin) "mist; cloud."

Neda: (Slavic) "Sunday's child."
Also: **Neda, Nedda, Nedi.**

Nedda: see Neda.

Neely: feminine form of Neal.

Neema: (Swahili) "bounty."

Neida: see Nerine.

Nelda: (Old English) "of the elder tree."
Also: **Nell.**

Nell, Nellie, Nelly: *see* Cornelia, Helen.

Neoma: (Greek) "the new moon."

Nereida, Nerida: *see* Nerine.

Neri, Neriah: "light, lamp of the Lord."

Nerine: (Greek) "nymph of the sea."
Also: **Neida, Nereen, Nereida, Nerida, Nerin, Nerina.**

Nerissa: (Greek) "of the sea." Literary: the delightful maid and companion to Portia in Shakespeare's *Merchant of Venice.*
Also: **Nerita.**

Nerys: (Welsh) "lord."

Nessa, Nessie: *see* Agnes.

Netta, Nettie: *see* Antonia, Natalie.

Neva: (Spanish) "extreme whiteness; snow."

Nevada: (Spanish) "white as snow."

Niabi: (American Indian) "a fawn."

Nichelle: combination of Nicole and Michelle.

Nicole: (Greek) "victory of the people." Feminine of Nicholas. Nicholassa Mohr, children's book author, illustrator.
Also: **Nichola, Nicola, Nicolette, Niki, Nikki, Nikola.**

Nicolette: variant of Nicole.

Nigella: (Latin) a flower name—love-in-a-mist.

Nikki: *see* Nicole. Nikki Giovanni, poet.

Nila: (Latin) "the River Nile of Egypt." Nila Mack, radio producer, writer.

Nina: (Spanish) "girl." Also a form of Ann.
Also: **Nina, Ninette, Ninita, Ninon.**

Ninita: (Spanish) "little girl."

Nissa: (Scandinavian) "a friendly elf."
Also: **Nissy, Nyssa.**

Nitsa: (Greek) "light."

Nixie: a water sprite of Germanic folklore.

Nobu: (NOH-boo) (Japanese) "faith." Nobu McCarthy, actress.
Also: **Nobuko.**

Noel: (Latin) "a Christmas child." Feminine of Noel.
Also: **Noella, Noelle.** *See also* Natalie.

Noelani: (Hawaiian) "mist; spray; the northeast trade wind; beautiful one from heaven."

Noelia: variant of Noel.

Noemi: Spanish form of Naomi.

Nokomis: (Chippewa Indian) "grandmother."

Nola: (Celtic) "famous; well-known." Feminine of Nolan.
Also: **Nolana.**

Noleta: (Latin) "unwilling."
Also: **Nolita.**

Noll, Nollie: *see* Olivia.

Nona: (Latin) "ninth-born."
Also: **Nonie, Nonna.**

Nora, Norah: *see* Helen,

Honora. Nora Ephron, writer.

Norberta: (Old German) "brilliant heroine." Feminine of Norbert.

Nordica: (German) "from the north."

Noreen, Norine, Norrie: *see* Honora.

Norma: (Latin) "the model." Feminine of Norman.
Also: **Normi, Normie.**

Norna: (Old Norse) a Viking goddess of fate.

Nova: (Latin) "new"; the name of a temporary star.

Novia: (Latin) "young person."
Also: **Nova.**

Nubia: (Latin) "Nubia."

Nunciata: (Latin) "announced; a messenger."
Also: **Annunciata, Nuncie.**

Nydia: (Latin) "a refuge."

Nyla: feminine form of Nyles.

Nyssa: (Greek) "starting point."
Also: **Nysa.**

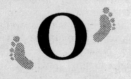

Obelia: (Greek) "a pillar."

Oceania: (Greek) "ocean."

Octavia: (Latin) "the eighth-born." Feminine of Octa-vius. Octavia, wife of Mark Antony.
Also: **Tavi, Tavia.**

Odele: (Greek) "a melody."
Also: **Odel, Odelet, Odell.**

Odelette: (French) "a little ode or lyric song."

Odelia: (Teutonic) "prosperous."
Also: **Odella, Odile.**

Odessa: (Greek) "a long journey." Odessa Komer, U.A.W. vice president.

Odette: (French) "home-lover; patriot." Odetta, folksinger.
Also: **Odet, Odetta.**

Ola: (Scandinavian) "daughter; descendant." Ola Winslow, author. Feminine of Olaf.

Olga: (Russian) "holy." Olga, first Russian saint of the Orthodox Church; Olga Korbut, Olympic gymnast.
Also: **Elga.**

Olinda: (Latin) "fragrant."

Olive: *see* Olivia. Olive Ann Beech, aircraft executive.

Olivia: (Latin) "the olive tree." The olive tree symbolizes fruitfulness, beauty, and dignity. Feminine of Oliver.
Also: **Liva, Livi, Livia, Livvi, Noll, Nollie, Olive, Olli, Ollie.**

Olympia: (Greek) "of the mountain of the gods." Olympia Brown, suffragette.
Also: **Olympe.**

Oma: (Arabic) "who has a long life." Feminine of Omar. Oma Barton, American union leader.

Ona, Oona: *see* Una.

Ondine: (Latin) "of water." Mythological water nymph of European tradition.
Also: **Undine.**

Oneida: (American Indian) "expected." The Oneida tribe, part of the Iroquois League, inhabited a region of central New York State.
Also: **Onida.**

Onyx: a jewel name.

Oona: *see* Una. Oona O'Neill, wife of Charlie Chaplin.

Opal: (Sanskrit) "jewel."

Ophelia: (Greek) "help." Literary: the tragic young girl in Shakespeare's *Hamlet.*
Also: **Opha, Phelia.**

Oprah: (Hebrew) "young deer." Oprah Winfrey, TV personality.
Also: **Ophrah, Orpah.**

Ora, Oralia, Oralie, Orel: *see* Aurelia.

Orah: (Israeli) "light."
Also: **Ora, Orly.**

Orela: (Latin) "a divine announcement."

Orenda: (Iroquois Indian) "magic power."

Oriana: (Latin) "the dawning; golden." Feminine of Orion.
Also: **Oralia.**

Oribel: (Latin) "of golden beauty."
Also: **Orabel, Orabelle, Ori, Oribelle.**

Oriole: (Latin) "fair; flaxen-haired."
Also: **Oriel.**

Orlena: (Latin) "the golden."
Also: **Orlene, Orlina.**

Orna: (Irish) "olive-colored."

Orpah: *see* Oprah.

Ortensia: (Latin) "a gardener." *See also* Hortense.

Orva: (Old English) "spear friend."

Osa: Osa Johnson, adventurer (1894–1953).

Ossia: feminine form of Ossian.

Ottilie: (Teutonic) "battle heroine." Tilly Edinger, paleontologist.
Also: **Otila, Otti, Ottie, Ottillia, Uta.**

Ozora: (Hebrew) "strength of the Lord."

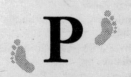

P

Pacifica: (Latin) "peaceable."

Paige: (Anglo-Saxon) "child; young."
Also: **Page.**

Pala: (Hawaiian) "fern." (American Indian) "water."

Paladia: (Latin) "protected by the goddess Pallas Athena." *See also* Pallas.

Palani: (Hawaiian) "sugarcane."

Pallas: (Greek) "wisdom, knowledge." Pallas Minerva, goddess of wisdom and war.
Also: **Palladia.**

Palma: (Latin) "palm tree."

Palmer: (Latin) "the palm-bearer; pilgrim."
Also: **Palma, Palmira.**

Paloma: (Spanish) "dove." Paloma Picasso, artist.
Also: **Palomita.**

Pamela: (origin uncertain) "loving; kind."
Also: **Pam, Pammy.**

Pandora: (Greek) "all-gifted." Mythology: when Pandora opened the box, she set free all evils upon humanity.
Also: **Dorie.**

Pano: (Hawaiian) "the color shiny black; deep blue-black."

Panphila: (Greek) "the all-loving one."

Pansy: (Greek) a flower name.
Also: **Pansie.**

Panthea: (Greek) "of all the gods."

Panya: a Russian form of Stephanie.

Paolina: variant of Paula.

Paris: a place name used as a contemporary first name.

Parker: (Middle English) "park keeper." Parker Posey, actress.

Parnella: (Old French) "little rock."
Also: **Pernella.**

Pascale: (French) "born at Easter."

Pat: see Patricia.

Patience: (Latin) "patient." A Puritan virtue name.

Patricia: (Latin) "of the nobility; wellborn." Feminine of Patrick. Pat Schroeder, congresswoman.
Also: **Pat, Patrice (Fr), Patrizia (It), Patsy, Patti, Patty, Tricia, Trish.**

Patsy: see Patricia.

Paula: (Latin) "little." Feminine of Paul. Pauline Trigere, designer.
Also: **Paolina, Paulette, Pauli, Paulie, Paulina, Pauline, Paulita.**

Paulina, Pauline: see Paula. Pauline Kael, film critic.

Payton: see Peyton.

Peace: (Latin) "tranquillity."

Pearl: (Latin) a jewel name. Also a form of Margaret. Pearl S. Buck, Nobel prize–winning author.
Also: **Pearla, Pearle, Pearline, Perl, Perle, Perlie.**

Peg, Peggy: familiar forms of Margaret.

Pegeen: (Celtic) "pearl."

Pelagia: (Greek) "from the sea."

Penelope: (Greek) "weaver." Mythology: the faithful wife of Odysseus who wove all day and unraveled her work at night.
Also: **Pen, Pennie, Penny.**

Penny: see Penelope. Penny Marshall, actress, director.

Penthea: (Greek) "mourner."

Peony: (Greek) a flower name.
Also: **Peonie.**

Pepita: (Spanish) "she shall add."
Also: **Pepi, Peta.**

Pepper: a contemporary nickname.

Perdita: (Latin) "lost." The name was created by Shakespeare for the heroine in *The Winter's Tale.*

Peregrine: (Latin) "traveler." Peregrine White was the first child born to English parents in New England. He was born on the *Mayflower* in Cape Cod Bay.
Also: **Perry.**

Perfecta: (Spanish) "perfect, accomplished one."

Perle: *see* Pearl.

Pernella: *see* Parnella.

Perry: (French) "pear tree." Perry Miller Adato, first woman to win an award from the Directors Guild of America (1977).
Also: **Perri, Perrie.**

Persephone: In Greek mythology, the beautiful daughter of Zeus and Demeter.

Persis: (Latin) "a woman from Persia." Persia Crawford Campbell, consumer advocate.

Petra: (Greek) "rock." A feminine form of Peter. Petra Barreras del Rio, art museum director; Petra Kelly, German political figure.
Also: **Peta, Pete, Petta.**

Petrina: (Greek) "steadfast; resolute." Another feminine form of Peter.
Also: **Petie, Petra, Petrine.**

Petula: (Latin) "saucy one."
Also: **Pet, Petulah.**

Petunia: (Latin) the petunia flower.

Peyton: (Latin) "noble; patrician."
Also: **Payton.**

Phedra: (Greek) "bright one."
Also: **Faydra, Phaedra, Phaidra.**

Phelia: *see* Ophelia.

Phenice: (Hebrew) "from a palm tree."
Also: **Phenica, Phenicia.**

Philana: (Greek) "friend of humankind."
Also: **Philina, Philine, Phillane.**

Philemena: *see* Philomena.

Philippa: (Greek) "lover of horses." Feminine of Philip.
Also: **Filipa, Philipa, Philippe, Pippa, Pippy.**

Philomena: (Greek) "loving friend."
Also: **Mena, Philemena, Philomene.**

Phoebe: (Greek) "the wise, shining one." Mythology: the daughter of Uranus and Gaea. Phoebe is the name of a Saturnian satellite. Phoebe Omlie, record-setting aviatrix.
Also: **Phebe.**

Phoenix: (Greek) "the heron or eagle." The phoenix was a mythological bird of ancient Egypt.

Phylicia: combination of Phyllis and Felicia. Phylicia Rashad, actress.

Phyllis: (Greek) "a green bough." Mythology Phyllis: a Thracian maiden who, despondent over her lover's absence, hangs herself and

turns into an almond tree. When her lover finally returns he embraces the almond tree, and the once barren plant puts forth new green leaves.
Also: **Philis, Phillis, Phyl, Phylis.**

Pia: (Italian) "devout." Pia Lindstrom, TV correspondent.

Pierrette: (French) "steady." Feminine of Pierre.

Pilar: (Spanish) "pillar."

Piper: (Old English) "a pipe player." Piper Laurie, actress.

Pippy: familiar form of Philippa.

Placida: (Latin) "gentle, peaceful one."
Also: **Placidia, Placilla.**

Platona: (Greek) feminine of Plato.

Pollock: (Old English) "little Paul."

Polly: *see* Mary.
Also: **Pol, Poll, Pollie.**

Pomona: (Latin) "fertile." Mythology: the Roman goddess of fruit trees.

Poppy: (Latin) a flower name. Poppy Cannon, food editor.

Portia: (Latin) a Roman family name whose root means "pig." Shakespeare introduced Portia in his plays *Julius Caesar* and *The Merchant of Venice.* Portia M. Hawkins Bond, *Essence* magazine.

Potter: (English) "a potter."

Precious: "of great value."
Also: **Preciosa.**

Prima: (Latin) "firstborn."

Primavera: (Spanish) "springtime."
Also: **Primalia.**

Primrose: (Latin) "the first rose."
Also: **Rose, Rosie.**

Priscilla: (Latin) "the ancient; of long lineage."
Also: **Cilla, Pris, Prisilla, Prissie, Prissy, Sil, Silla.**

Priya: (Sanskrit) "beloved; darling."

Prospera: (Latin) "favorable."
Also: **Prosper.**

Prudence: (Latin) "the prudent; cautious."
Also: **Pru, Prudencia, Prudentia, Prudi, Prudie, Prudy.**

Prunella: (French) "plum tree."
Also: **Pru, Prue, Nell, Nellie.**

Psyche: (Greek) "the soul." Mythology: a beautiful maiden who won the love of Cupid.

Purity: (English) "purity."

Pyrena: (Greek) "fiery one."

Pythia: (Greek) "a prophet."

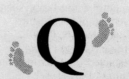

Q

Qian: (Chinese) "pretty; courteous."
Also: **Qian Lin.**

Queena: (Teutonic) "a queen; a woman."

Queenie: see Regina.

Quenby: (Scandinavian) "wife; womanly."

Querida: (Spanish) "loved one."

Quinn: (Gaelic) "wise and intelligent."

Quinta: (Latin) "the fifth child." Feminine of Quinton.
Also: **Quintina.**

Quirita: (Latin) "citizen."

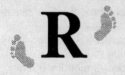

R

Rabi: (Arabic) "spring; harvest."

Rachel: (Hebrew) "naive and innocent; like a lamb." The biblical Rachel was "beautiful and well favored" and dearly loved by her husband Jacob. Rachel Carson, writer.
Also: **Rachele, Rachelle, Rae, Raquel (Sp), Ray, Rochelle, Shelley.**

Radella: (Old English) "elfin counselor."

Radha: (Hindustani) "golden bloom of the garden of heaven."

Radinka: (Slavic) "active one."

Radmilla: (Slavic) "worker for the people."

Rae, Ray: see Rachel. Ray Kaiser Eames, designer.

Rahima: (Swahili) "compassionate."
Also: **Rahiima.**

Rain: the English word used as a first name. Rain, daughter of comedian Richard Pryor.

Rainbow: the English word used as a first name.

Raine: (French) "queen."
Also: **Rayna, Rayne, Reine.**

Raissa: (Old French) "thinker, believer."

Ramona: (Teutonic) "protector." Feminine of Raymond.
Also: **Mona, Rama.**

Rana: (Sanskrit) "of royalty."
Also: **Rani, Rania.**

Randy: short form of Miranda. Randye Sandel, artist.
Also: **Randee, Randi.**

Raphaela: (Hebrew) "blessed healer." Feminine of Raphael.
Also: **Rafaela.**

Raquel, Raquelle: Spanish forms of Rachel. Raquel Welch, actress.

Rashida: (Arabic) "intelligent."

Raven: (English) a bird name; a recurring hero in the mythology of Indian tribes of the Pacific Northwest coast.

Ray-: short form of names beginning Ra-. Ray (Rachel) Strachey, English feminist.

Rayha: (Swahili) "small comfort."

Reba: short form of Rebecca.

Reba McEntire, country singer.

Rebecca: (Hebrew) "the captivator." Biblical: the mother of Esau and Jacob, the founder of the house of Israel. Rebecca West, author.
Also: **Becka, Becky, Reba, Rebekah, Riba, Riva.**

Reed: (English) "red-haired."
Also: **Read, Reid.**

Regan: (Teutonic) "pertaining to royalty."

Regina: (Latin) "queen." Regina Belle, pop singer.
Also: **Gina, Gine, Queenie, Regan, Reggie, Regine.** *See also* Raine.

Reiko: (RAY-koh) (Japanese) "clear, beautiful child." Rei Kawakubo, fashion designer.

Reilly: *see* Riley.

Remy: (French) "from Rheims."

Ren: (Japanese) "water lily."

Rena: *see* Irene.

Renata: (Latin) "reborn." Renata Adler, writer.

Renee, Rennae: (French) "reborn." Rennae Stubbs, tennis player.
Also: **Renata, Reni, Rennie.**

Reseda: (Latin) "the mignonette flower."

Reva: (Latin) "to regain strength."

Rexana: (Latin-English) "regally graceful."

Rhea: (Greek) "a stream." Mythological: daughter of heaven and earth, mother of the great gods. Rhea Seddon, U.S. astronaut.

Rhianna: (Muslim) "sweet basil."
Also: **Riana, Rihana.**

Rhiannon: (Welsh) "nymph goddess." Mythology: an ancient Celtic goddess.

Rhoda: (Greek) "a garland of roses."
Also: **Rodi, Rodie.**

Rhodanthe: (Greek) "rose flower."

Rhodia: *see* Rose.

Ria: (Spanish) "a river mouth."

Ricadonna: (English-Italian) "ruling lady."

Ricarda: (Old English) feminine of Richard.

Ricky: diminutive of Erica, Frederica and Ricarda.

Riley: the Irish surname used as a first name.
Also: **Reilly.**

Rilla: (Low German) "a stream or brook."

Rima: (Spanish) "poetry."

Rinnah: (Hebrew) "full of joy."
Also: **Rinah.**

Ripley: (Old English) "dweller at the shouter's meadow."

Risa: (Latin) "laughter."
Also: **Rise.**

Rita: (Greek) "a pearl." A diminutive of Clarita, Margarita, and Norita, but also used as an independent name. Rita Mae Brown, feminist, writer.

Riva: *see* Rebecca.

Roanna: (Latin) "sweet; gracious."
Also: **Roana, Roanne.**

Roberta: (Anglo-Saxon) "of shining fame." Feminine of Robert. Roberta Flack, singer, songwriter.
Also: **Robbie, Robina, Ruberta, Ruperta.** *See also* Robin.

Robin: (English) the robin bird. Also a familiar form of Roberta.
Also: **Bobbie, Bobby, Robbie, Robby, Robyn.**

Rochana: (Persian) "dawn of day."

Rochelle: *see* Rachel.
Also: **Shelley, Shelly.**

Rolanda: (Old German) "famous land."
Also: **Rolande.**

Roma: (Latin) Italian name of the city of Rome.
Also: **Romy.**

Romana: (Latin) a form of Roma. Romana Acosta Banuelos, former U.S. treasurer; Romaine Brooks, artist.

Romy: *see* Rosemary.

Rona: a Scottish place name.
Also: **Rhona, Ronny.**

Ronnie: short form of Veronica. Also an independent name.

Rosalie: a form of Rose.
Also: **Rosaleen, Rozalie.**

Rosalind: (Latin) "beautiful rose." Rosalynn Carter, First Lady of the U.S.
Also: **Rosaleen, Rosalinda, Rosaline, Rosalynd.** *See also* Rose, Roselyn.

Rosamund: (Latin) "rose of the world."

Rosangela: combination of Rose and Angela. Rosangela Renno, artist.

Rosanna: variant of Rose. Rosanna Arquette, actress.

Rose: (Latin) "a rose." Rose Bird, chief justice of the California Supreme Court; Rosa Parks, civil rights figure.
Also: **Rhodia, Rosa, Rosalee, Rosaleen, Rosalia, Rosalie, Rosamond, Rosamund, Rosanna, Rosel, Rosella, Roselle, Rosena, Rosetta, Rosette, Rosie, Rosina, Rosita, Rossene, Rozalie, Rozina.** *See also* Primrose.

Roseanne: variant of Rose.

Roselyn: a popular form of Rosalind.
Also: **Rosalyn, Roslyn, Roz.**

Rosemary: (Latin) "Mary's rose"; the fragrant herb.
Also: **Romy, Rosemarie.**

Rosena: *see* Rose.

Rowan: (Irish) "little red one; rowan tree."
Also: **Rowann, Rowanne.**

Rowena: (Celtic) "flowing white hair." The Saxon maiden in Sir Walter Scott's *Ivanhoe* (1819).
Also: **Rhonwen (Welsh), Rowe.**

Roxanne: (Persian) "dawn." Roxane, love interest of the hero Cyrano de Bergerac in the Rostand play.
Also: **Rox, Roxana, Roxane, Roxanna, Roxanne, Roxie, Roxy.**

Roxy: *see* Roxanne.

Royale: (Old French) feminine of Roy.

Ruby: (Latin) a jewel. Ruby Dee, actress.
Also: **Rubi, Rubie.**

Rudelle: (Old German) "famous one."
Also: **Rudella.**

Rudi, Rudy: feminine of Rudolph.

Rue: a botanical name. Rue McClanahan, TV actress.

Rufina: (Latin) feminine of Rufus.

Rumer: (English) "gypsy." Rumer Godden, British novelist.

Ruth: (Hebrew) "a beautiful friend." Biblical: the Book of Ruth. Ruth Prawer Jhabvala, novelist, screenwriter.
Also: **Ruthie.**

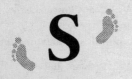

Saba: (Greek) "woman of Sheba."

Sabina: (Latin) "Sabine woman." Sabine Appelmans, tennis player.
Also: **Sabine, Savina.**

Sable: (Slavic) "black"; a valuable fur.

Sabra: (Hebrew) "thorny." Name given to a native-born Israeli girl. (Arabic) "patience."

Sabrina: (Anglo-Saxon) "a princess." *Sabrina,* the romantic comedy film (1954, 1995).
Also: **Brina, Zabrina.**

Sacha: (Greek) "helper."

Sachi: (Hindi) wife of Indra.

Sachiko: (SAH-chee-koh) (Japanese) "good fortune, happiness, child."
Also: **Sachi.**

Sade: (shar-DAY) Popularized by the contemporary singer Sade.

Sadie, Sadye: *see* Sarah.

Sadira: (Persian) "the lotus tree."

Sadybeth: combination of Sadie/Sady and Beth.

Saffron: (Arabic) "the crocus flower."

Sage: (English-French) "wise one"; a name from nature.

Sahara: (Arabic) "wilderness." (Hebrew) "moon." The Sahara, covering an area the size of the U.S., is the world's largest desert.
Also: **Sahra.**

Salama: *see* Salem.

Salem: (Arabic) "complete, perfect peace."
Also: **Salima.**

Salena: (Greek) "salty."
Also: **Salina.**

Salima: *see* Salem.

Sallie, Sally: *see* Sarah. Sally Ride, first American woman in space.

Salome: (Hebrew) "a woman of perfection." (Arabic) "safe."

Salvia: (Latin) "sage."
Also: **Salvina.**

Samantha: a feminine form of Samuel.
Also: **Sam, Sami, Sammy.**

Samara: (Hebrew) "watchful; cautious."
Also: **Mara.**

Samuela: (Hebrew) "name of God." Feminine of Samuel.
Also: **Sam, Samella, Samuelia.**

Sancia: (Latin) "sacred."
Also: **Sanchia.**

Sandra, Sandy: short forms of Alexandra. Sandra Day O'Connor, Supreme Court justice.

Sandrine, Sandrina: forms of Sandra.

Santana: (Spanish) "Saint Anna/Anne."

Santina: (Latin) "little saint."
Also: **Santa.**

Sapphire: (Greek) a jewel name.
Also: **Sapphira.**

Sarah: (Hebrew) "princess." Biblical: the wife of Abraham.
Also: **Sada, Sadie, Sadye, Sal, Sallie, Sally, Sara, Sarena, Sarene, Saretta, Sari, Sarita, Shari, Sharon, Zara.**

Saretta, Sarita: see Sarah. Sarita Choudhury, actress.

Sasha: a Russian form of Alexandra.
Also: **Sacha, Sascha.**

Saskia: (Dutch) "Saxon woman." The name of Rembrandt's wife, who was the subject of some of his notable portraits.

Savannah: (Spanish) "a grassland"; the picturesque Georgia city.
Also: **Savanna.**

Savita: (Hindi) "sun."

Scarlett: (English-French) the bright red color. Popularized as a name by Scarlett O'Hara, heroine of *Gone with the Wind.* Elizabeth Scarlett Jagger, child of rock star Mick Jagger and Jerry Hall.

Schifra: (Hebrew) "beautiful."
Also: **Shifrah.**

Scientia: (Latin) "to know."

Seana: feminine of Sean.
Also: **Sean, Seanna, Shawn.**

Season: (Latin) "time of sowing." Season Hubley, actress.

Sebastiane: (Latin) feminine of Sebastian.
Also: **Sebastianna.**

Secunda: (Latin) "second child."

Sela: see Sheila. Sela Ward, actress.

Selena: (Greek) name derived from Selene, the Greek moon goddess.
Also: **Celine, Lena, Salene.**

Selma: (Celtic) "the fair." Selma Lagerlöf, first woman to win the Nobel prize for literature. *See also* Anselma.

Semele: (Latin) "a single time."

Semira: (Hebrew) "the height of the heavens."

Septima: (Latin) "seventh child."

Seraphina: (Hebrew) "burning or ardent one."
Also: **Sera, Serafina, Serafine, Seraphine.**

Serena: (Latin) "tranquil."
Also: **Serene, Serenity.**

Sevilla: (Latin) a place name.

Shaina: (Hebrew) "beautiful."
Also: **Shaine, Shayna.**

Shakira: (Arabic) "thankful."

Shan: (Chinese) "coral; mountain." A prefix often combined with another name.

Shana: (Irish) "wise." Shana Alexander, journalist.

Shane: a form of John. Shane Gould, Australian swimmer.

Shani: (SHAH-nee) (Hebrew) "scarlet; crimson."

Shannon: (Irish Gaelic) a place name referring to the longest river in Ireland. Shannon Lucid, U.S. astronaut.
Also: **Shana, Shandy, Shani, Shannah, Shannen, Shanon, Shauna, Shawna.**

Shantal: *see* Chantal.

Shantay: a contemporary name from Shante, Sanskrit word meaning peaceful.
Also: **Shanti.**

Shanti: *see* Shantay.

Shari: variant of Sarah and Sharon.

Sharmila: (Sanskrit) "modest."

Sharon: (Hebrew) "of the land of Sharon."
Also: **Shara, Shari, Sharona, Sherry.** *See also* Sarah.

Shawana: (Swahili) "grace."

Shawn: variant of Sean (John) used as a female name.
Also: **Sean, Shawna.**

Shawnee: (American Indian) "southerners." Shawnee Pickney, basketball player.

Sheba: *see* Bathsheba.

Sheena: a Scottish form of Jane. Sheena Easton, singer, actress.

Sheila: (Celtic) "musical."
Also: **Seela, Sela, Sheela, Shelaugh, Shelley, Shielah.** *See also* Cecilia.

Shelby: (English) "willow farm." Shelby Woo, television character.

Shelley: (English) "meadow on the ledge."
Also: **Shellie, Shelly.** *See also* Rachel, Sheila.

Sheridan: the Irish surname traditionally used as a boy's first name.
Also: **Sherry.**

Sherilyn: variant of Cheryl. Sherilyn Fenn, actress.
Also: **Sheralyn.**

Sheri, Sherry: *see* Cherie, Shirley. Sherry Lansing, film executive.

Sheryl: *see* Cheryl.

Shifra: *see* Schifra.

Shiloh: (Hebrew) "peace, abundance."

Shimona: (Hebrew) feminine of Shimon.

Shirley: (Anglo-Saxon) "from the white meadow." Shirley Temple Black, child actress, U.S. ambassador.

Also: **Sheri, Sherry, Shirl, Shirlee, Shirlene, Shirlie.**

Shita: (Hebrew) the acacia tree.

Shoshanna: a Hebrew form of Susan, Susanna.

Sian: a Welsh form of Jane.
Also: **Siana.**

Sibyl: *see* Sybil.

Sidney: *see* Sydney.

Sidonia: (Latin) "a woman from Sidon."
Also: **Sidonie, Sydney.**

Sienna: (Latin) "from Sienna."

Sierra: (Latin) "saw-toothed mountain." A mountain range in California.

Sigfreda: (Old German) "victorious and peaceful."

Signa: (Latin) "a signer."

Sigourney: (French) "daring king." Sigourney Weaver, actress.

Sigrid: (Old Norse) "victorious counselor." Sigrid Undset, Nobel prize–winning Norwegian author.

Silvana: *see* Sylvia.

Silvia: *see* Sylvia.

Simone: (Hebrew) "heard by the Lord." Simone Weil, French philosopher.
Also: **Simona, Simonne.**

Sinéad: (Irish Gaelic) variant of Jane. Sinéad O'Connor, rock singer.

Sissy: variant of Jane. Sissy Spacek, actress.

Sister: an American nickname. Sister Parish, interior designer.

Sky, Skye: the English word.

Skylar, Skyler: (Dutch) "sheltering."
Also: **Sky, Skye.**

Sofia: Spanish and Italian form of Sophia.

Solana: (Spanish) "sunshine."

Soledad: (Spanish) "solitude."

Solita: (Latin) "solitary."
Also: **Sola, Soledad.**

Soloma: (Persian) "peaceable."

Solvig: (Old German) "victorious battle maid."

Sondra: *see* Alexandra.

Sonia, Sonja, Sonya: Scandinavian and Slavic form of Sophie. Sonia Delaunay, artist; Sonja Henie, skater.

Sonora: the province in Mexico.

Sophie/Sophia: (Greek) "wisdom." Sophia Loren, actress.
Also: **Sofia (Sp, It), Sonia, Sonja, Sonya, Sophey, Sophie (Fr), Sophy, Zofia (Pol).**

Sorcha: (Irish) "bright."

Sorrel: (origin uncertain) a plant name and the name of a reddish-brown color.
Also: **Sorell, Sorrel.**

Spring: (Old English) "springtime." Spring Byington, actress.

Stacy, Stacey: *see* Anastasia.
Also: **Staci, Stacie.**

Starr: (Anglo-Saxon) "star."
Also: **Star.**

Stella: a short form of Estelle. Stella Adler, acting teacher.

Stephanie: (Greek) "a crown;

garland." Feminine of Stephen. Steffi Graf, tennis player.
Also: **Panya, Stefanie, Steffie, Stephana, Stephania, Stephenie, Stevie.**

Stevie: feminine of Stephen. Stevie Smith, poet; Stevie Nicks, rock singer.

Stockard: (English) "from the field of tree stumps." Stockard Channing, actress.

Storm: (Old English) "a tempest or storm."
Also: **Stormy.**

Sufa: (Hebrew) "storm"; an Israeli place name.

Sukie, Sukey: pet forms of Susan.

Sullivan: (Irish Gaelic) "black-eyed one."

Sumi: (SOO-mee) (Japanese) "joyous; beautiful."

Summer: (English) "summer." Summer Sanders, swimmer.

Sumner: (Latin) "the summoner."

Sunny: (English) "bright; genial."
Also: **Sun.**

Surya: (Hindi) "sun god." Surya Bonaly, skater.

Susan: (Hebrew) "a lily." Susan B. Anthony, women's rights activist.
Also: **Shoshana, Sue, Sukey, Sukie, Susana, Susanna, Susannah, Susanne, Susi, Susie, Susy, Suzanna, Suzette, Suzie, Suzy, Zuzanna (Pol).**

Susanna, Susannah: variants of Susan.

Svetlana: (Slavic) "light." Svetlana Savitskaya, Soviet cosmonaut.

Sybil: (Greek) "the prophetess."
Also: **Cybil, Sib, Sibbie, Sibby, Sibel, Sibell, Sibie, Sibyl, Sybyl.**

Sydel: (Hebrew) "the enchantress."
Also: **Sydelle.**

Sydney: (Hebrew) "the enticer." Feminine of Sidney. Sydne Vogel, ice skater.
Also: **Cidney, Cydney, Sid, Sidney, Sidonia, Sidonie, Syd, Sydny.**

Sylvia: (Latin) "forest maiden." Sylvia Beach, publisher; Sylvia Plath, poet.
Also: **Silva, Silvana, Silvia, Syl, Sylvie.**

Sylviane: variant of Sylvia. Sylviane Puntous, triathlete.

Syna: (Greek) "together."

Synthia, Sindy: *see* Cynthia.

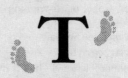

Tabitha: (Aramaic) "the gazelle." Tabitha Soren, TV correspondent.
Also: **Tabbie, Tabita.**

Tabor: (Hebrew) "purity."

Tacita: (Latin) "silent."
Also: **Tacy.**

Taffy: (Welsh) "beloved."

Tal: (Hebrew) "dew."
Also: **Tali, Talila, Talya.**

Talassi: (American Indian) "corn tassel flower."

Talia: (Hebrew) "lamb." Talia Shire, actress.
Also: **Talie, Tally.**

Talitha: (Aramaic) "maiden."
Also: **Talita, Tally.**

Tallulah: (American Indian) "leaping water." Tallulah Bankhead, actress.
Also: **Tallu, Tallula.**

Tama: (American Indian) "thunderbolt."

Tamara: (Hebrew) "the palm tree." Biblical: daughter of King David. Tamara McKinney, skier.
Also: **Tamar.**

Tameron: an invented name.

Tamiko: (tah-MEE-koh) (Japanese): "the people."
Also: **Tami, Tammy.**

Tamlyn: a contemporary name. Tamlyn Tomita, actress.

Tammy: a familiar form of Tamara and other names beginning Tam-.

Tamsen, Tamsin, Tamson: feminine of Thomasina.

Tangerine: (English) "girl from the city of Tangier."
Also: **Tangier.**

Tania: *see* Tanya.

Tanith: the Phoenician goddess Tanith was known to the Greeks as Artemis and to the Romans as Diana.

Tanner: (Old English) "leather maker."

Tansy: (Middle Latin) "tenacious one"; a flower name.

Tanya: (Slavic) meaning unknown. Tanya Tucker, country singer.
Also: **Tania, Tanja.**

Tao: (Chinese) "peach." A prefix often combined with another name.

Tara: (Celtic) "tower." In Irish legend, Tara is the home of ancient Irish kings. Tara Fitzgerald, actress.

Taryn: a contemporary combination of Tara and Erin.
Also: **Tarin, Tarryn, Teryn.**

Tasha: a pet form of Natasha.

Taslima: Taslima Nasrin, Bangladeshi writer.

Tate: *see* Tatum.

Tatiana, Tatyana: (Russian) Tatyana Samolenko, track athlete.
Also: **Tatijana, Tatyana.**

Tatum: (English) "cheerful." Tatum O'Neal, actress.
Also: **Tate.**

Taura: (English) feminine form of Taurus. Taurus the Bull is a constellation of the zodiac.

Tavia: *see* Octavia.

Tawny: (Irish) "a green field"; the sandy color, as in the color of a lion's coat. Tahnee Welch, actress.
Also: **Tawnee, Tawney, Tawnya.**

Taylor: (Middle English) "a tailor." Taylor Caldwell, author.
Also: **Tailor.**

Teddi, Teddie: short forms of Theodora.

Teena: short form of Christine and Ernestine.

Temperance: a Puritan virtue name.

Tempest: (Old French) "stormy one."

Tenley: (origin uncertain) Tenley Albright, champion figure skater.

Terentia: (Greek) "guardian."

Teresa: (Greek) "the harvester." The name of two popular saints, Teresa of Avila and Therese of Lisieux. Mother Teresa, winner of the Nobel Peace Prize.
Also: **Terese, Teressa, Teri, Terrie, Terry, Tess, Tessa, Tessie, Theresa, Therese (Fr), Tracey, Tracy, Tressa, Zita.**

Teri: see Teresa.

Terra: (Latin) "the earth."
Also: **Terrah, Tierra.**

Terry: see Teresa.

Tesia: (Polish) "loved by God."

Tess: short form of Teresa. Literary: title character of the Thomas Hardy novel *Tess of the d'Urbervilles. See also* Teresa, Tessa.

Tessa: (Greek) "fourth child." Tessa Martinez Tagle, college president.
Also: **Tess, Tessie.**

Thaddea: (Greek) "courageous one."

Thai Binh: (Vietnamese) "peace." Thai Ishizuka Capp, student.

Thalia: (Greek) "blooming." Mythology: the Greek goddess of comedy and poetry.

Thandie: (Zulu) "loved one." Thandie Newton, actress.

Thea: (Greek) "goddess." Thea Musgrave, British conductor, composer.
Also: **Theia.** *See also* Alethea, Althea, Anthea, Theodora.

Theano: (Greek) "divine name."

Thecla: (Greek) "divinely famous."
Also: **Thekla.**

Theda: see Theodora. Theda Bara, actress.

Thelma: (Greek) "nursing." Thelma Cooke, executive at Anheuser-Busch.

Theo: see Theodora, Theola.

Theodora: (Greek) "God's divine gift." A feminine form of Theodore.
Also: **Dora, Dori, Teddi, Teddie, Teodora (It, Sp), Thea, Theda, Theo, Theodosia, Thia.**

Theola: (Greek) "heaven-sent."
Also: **Lola, Theo.**

Thera: (Greek) "untamed."

Theresa: see Teresa.

Thetis: (Greek) "positive, determined one." The mother of Achilles.

Thirza: (Hebrew) "pleasant-ness."

Thomasina: (Hebrew) "the twin." Feminine of Thomas.
Also: **Tamsen, Thomasa, Thomasine, Tomasina, Tomie, Tommie, Tommy.**

Thora: (Teutonic) "thunder."

Thordis: (Old Norse) "Thor-spirit."

Thulani: (origin uncertain) Thulani Davis, poet, playwright.

Thyra: (Greek) "shield bearer."

Tia: a contemporary name (Spanish for aunt or Egyptian for princess, sister of King Ramses.)

Tian: (Tee-AHN) (Chinese) "heaven; tranquil; sweet." Traditionally combined with a second name.

Tiara: (Latin) "headdress."

Tiberia: (Latin) "of the River Tibes." Tiberia Mitri, soap opera actress.

Tierney: (Irish Gaelic) "lordly one." Tierney Sutton, singer.
Also: **Tiernan.**

Tifara: (Hebrew) "beauty; splendor."

Tiffany: (Greek) "appearance of God."
Also: **Tiffani.**

Tilda, Tillie, Tilly: *see* Mathilda.

Timothea: (Greek) "honoring God." Feminine of Timothy.
Also: **Timmy.**

Tina: diminutive of Christine, Ernestine, and Martina, but also used as an independent name. Tina Brown, magazine editor.

Tipper: (Irish) nickname and variant of Tabar, an Irish name meaning "well."

Tippi, Tippie: *see* Zipporah.

Tira: (Hebrew) "villa; small village."

Tita: (Latin) "a title of honor."

Titania: (Greek) "giant."
Also: **Tania.**

Toby, Tobey: (Hebrew) "God is good." Feminine of Tobias.
Also: **Tobe, Tobi.**

Toni, Tony: *see* Antonia. Toni Morrison, Nobel prize–winning novelist.

Tonya: (Russian) short form of Antonia, Latonia.

Topaz: (Latin) "a topaz gem."

Tori, Tory: (Scottish/English) Diminutive of Victoria. Tori Amos, singer.
Also: **Toriana, Torrey, Torri, Torrie, Torry.**

Torrey, Torry: a Scottish place name.

Tosca: (Latin) "from Tuscany."

Toshiko: (Japanese) "superior; intelligent." Toshiko Akiyoshi, jazz composer.

Tovah: (Hebrew) "good." Tovah Feldshuh, actress.
Also: **Tova, Tovit.**

Tracy: *see* Teresa.

Traviata: (Italian) "one who goes astray."

Trella: (TREH-yuh) (Spanish) "little star." A diminutive of Estrella.

Tricia: familiar form of Patricia.

Trilby: (uncertain origin) "frivolous; giddy." Trilby O'Ferral, young model seduced by the sinister Svengali in novel *Trilby* (1894).

Trina: short form of names ending -trina.

Trinity: (Latin) "triad." The

Holy Trinity. Trini Alvarado, actress.
Also: **Trinidad.**

Trish, Trisha: familiar form of Patricia. Trisha Brown, choreographer.
Also: **Tisha.**

Trista: (Latin) "woman of sadness." Feminine of Tristan.
Also: **Tristana.**

Trixie: see Beatrice.

Trudy: see Gertrude.

True: (Old English) "faithful, loyal one."
Also: **Truly.**

Tsiporah: see Zipporah.

Tuesday: (Old English) "born on Tuesday." Tuesday Weld, actress.

Tullia: (Irish Gaelic) "peaceful, quiet one."
Also: **Tulie, Tully.**

Tuwa: (Hopi Indian) "earth."

Twyla: (Middle English) "woven of double thread." Twyla Tharp, dancer.
Also: **Twila.**

Tyne: (Old English) "river." Tyne Daly, actress.
Also: **Tyna.**

Tyra: (Scandinavian) "of Tyr, god of battle." Tyra Banks, model.

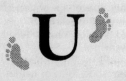

Ualani: (Hawaiian) "heavenly rain."

Uda: (Old German) "prosperous one."

Udele: (Anglo-Saxon) "woman of great wealth."

Ula: (Celtic) "sea jewel." See also Ullah.

Ulima: (Arabic) "wise, learned one."

Ullah: (Hebrew) "a burden."

Ulma: (Latin) "the elm tree."

Ulrica: (Teutonic) "ruler of all." Feminine of Ulric. Ulrike Meyfarth, German Olympic gold medalist in track.
Also: **Rica, Ulrika.**

Ultima: (Latin) "aloof one."

Ulva: (Gothic) "wolf."

Uma: (OO-mah) (Hindustani) "mother; wife of Shiva." Uma Thurman, actress.

Umeko: (oo-MEH-koh) (Japanese) "plum blossom."

Umi: (Swahili) "my mother."

Una: (Latin) "all truth is one." Character in the Edmund Spenser verse romance *The Faerie Queene.*
Also: **Ona, Oona.**

Undine: (Latin) "of water."
Also: **Undina.** See also Ondine.

Unity: (English) "unity."

Urania: (Greek) "heavenly."
Also: **Uranie.**

Urbana: (Latin) "of the city."

Uria, Uriela: (Hebrew) "light of God." A symbolic name for girls born on Hanukkah.
Also: **Uriah.**

Ursula: (Latin) "she-bear." St. Ursula.

Also: **Ursa, Ursel, Ursi, Ursulette.**

Uta: *see* Ottilie.

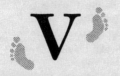

Vail: (Anglo-Saxon) "from the valley."

Vala: (Gothic) "chosen one."

Valda: (Teutonic) "battle heroine."
Also: **Val.**

Valencia: *see* Valentina.

Valentina: (Latin) "the vigorous and strong." Feminine of Valentine. Valentina Tereshkova, first woman to travel in space.
Also: **Val, Valencia, Valentia, Valeria, Valerie, Vallie, Valora.**

Valerie: *see* Valentina.

Valonia: (Latin) "from the vale."

Vanda: Slavic form of Wanda.

Vanessa: a name invented in the 18th century by Jonathan Swift.
Also: **Nessa, Van, Vanni.**

Vania: (Hebrew) "God's gracious gift." A feminine form of John.
Also: **Van.**

Vanna: variant of Vanessa.

Vanora: (Old Welsh) "white wave."

Varda: (Hebrew) "rose-colored; pink."
Also: **Vardiella, Vardina, Vardis.**

Varsha: (Hindi) "rain."

Vashti: (Hebrew) "fairest, loveliest woman." Biblical: wife of the Persian king Xerxes.
Also: **Vashta, Vasti.**

Veda: (Sanskrit) "wise."

Vega: (Arabic) "the falling one."

Velda: (Teutonic) "of great wisdom."
Also: **Valeda.**

Velma: *see* Wilhelmina.

Velvet: (Middle English) "velvety." Velvet Brown, heroine of *National Velvet*.

Vemtira: (Spanish) "happiness and good luck."

Venetia: (Latin) "blessed"; the Latin form of Venice.
Also: **Venicia.**

Venus: (Latin) "loveliness." Ancient goddess later associated with the Greek goddess of love, Aphrodite. Venus Williams, tennis player.
Also: **Venetia.**

Vera: (Latin) "true."
Also: **Veradis, Verine.**

Verda: (Latin) "young and fresh."
Also: **Verdie.**

Vern: *see* Laverne.

Verna: (Latin) "spring-born." Feminine of Vernon.
Also: **Vernice, Vernita.** *See also* Laverne.

Veronica: (Latin) "true image."
Also: **Ronnie, Ronny, Veronique, Vonny.**

Vespera: (Latin) "the evening star."

Vesta: (Latin) "guardian of the sacred fire; vestal virgin." Mythology: Roman goddess of the hearth.
Also: **Esta.**

Vevila: (Irish Gaelic) "melodious, harmonious lady."

Vicki, Vicky: *see* Victoria.

Victoria: (Latin) "the victorious." Feminine of Victor. Victoria, queen of England, the longest-reigning monarch in English history.
Also: **Tori, Torry, Vicki, Vicky, Victorie, Victorine, Vittoria (It).**

Vida: (Hebrew) "beloved one."
Also: **Davida, Veda, Vita.**

Vignette: (French) "little vine."

Villa: (Latin) "a country estate."

Vilma: (Russian) "protector."

Vinna: (Anglo-Saxon) "of the vine."
Also: **Vina, Vine.**

Viola: *see* Violet.

Violet: (Latin) the violet flower.
Also: **Vi, Viola, Violetta, Violette, Wioletta (Polish).**

Viona: *see* Fionna.

Virginia: (Latin) "maidenly; pure." Virginia Apgar, physician.
Also: **Ginger, Ginny, Jinny, Virgilia, Virginie, Virgy.**

Viridiana: (Latin) "green." An Italian saint's name.

Virtue: (Latin) moral goodness; one of the Puritan virtue names.

Vita: (Latin) "life." Vita Sackville-West, writer.
Also: **Vitala.**

Viva: (Latin) "full of life." Viveka Davis, actress.
Also: **Viveca.**

Vivian: (Latin) "lovely; full of life."
Also: **Vi, Viv, Vivi, Vivia, Viviane, Vivie, Vivien, Vivienne.**

Volante: (Italian) "flying one."

Voleta: (Old French) "a flowing veil."

Vondra: (Czech) "brave."

Vonnie, Vonny: *see* Veronica, Yvonne.

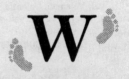

W

Wallis: (Teutonic) "girl of Wales." Wallis Warfield, duchess of Windsor.
Also: **Walli, Wallie, Wally.**

Wanda: (Teutonic) "the wanderer."
Also: **Wenda.**

Wanetta: (Old English) "pale one."

Warda: (Old German) feminine of Ward.

Waverly: (Old English) "quaking-aspen-tree meadow."

Wei: (Chinese) "small, slight; rose." A prefix often combined with another name.

Welcome: (English) "a welcome guest."

Wendy: a name first used by J. M. Barrie in *Peter Pan*. Wendy Wasserstein, dramatist.
Also: **Wende, Wendie.** *See also* Gwendolen.

Wenona: *see* Winona.

Wesley: traditionally a boy's name. Weslia Whitfield, singer.

Whitley: (English) "white meadow."

Whitney: (English) "fair island." Whitney Houston, singer.

Wilda: (Anglo-Saxon) "the untamed; the wild one."

Wilfreda: (Teutonic) "firm peacemaker." Feminine of Wilfred.
Also: **Freda, Freddie.**

Wilhelmina: (Teutonic) "protectress." Wilhelmina, queen of the Netherlands.
Also: **Mina, Velma, Wilma.**

Willa: (Anglo-Saxon) "desirable." Feminine of William. Willa Cather, author.

Willamae: combination of Willa and Mae.

Willow: a contemporary name from nature.

Wilma: *see* Wilhelmina. Wilma Mankiller, first

woman deputy chief of the Five Tribes Organization.

Winema: (Modoc Indian) "woman chief."

Winifred: (Teutonic) "friend of peace."
Also: **Freddie, Winnie, Winny.**

Winnie, Winny: familiar forms of Edwina, Winifred, Winona, Wynne.

Winona: (American Indian) "the firstborn." Winona Ryder, actress.
Also: **Wenona, Wenonah, Win, Winny, Wynonna.**

Winter: (Old English) "winter."

Wioletta: (Polish) "violet."

Wren: (Welsh) "chief"; the wren bird.

Wynne: (Celtic) "the fair; the white."
Also: **Winne, Winnie, Winny, Wyne.**

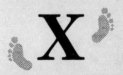

Xandra, Xandrine: forms of Alexandra.

Xanthe: (Greek) "blond."

Xaviera: (Spanish) "owner of the new house."

Xena: (Greek) "hospitable."
Also: **Xenia, Zenia.**

Xian: (Chinese) "celebrated; celestial being; brightly colored." Traditionally combined with a second name.

Ximena: uncertain origin; possible Basque.

Xina: *see* Christine.

Xylia: (Greek) "of the wood."

Xylina: (Greek) "wood dweller."

Xyloma: (Greek) "from the forest."

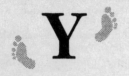

Yafa: (YAH-fah) (Hebrew) "lovely"; an Israeli place name.

Yamilla: (Arabic) "beautiful." Yamila Azize, academic.

Yan: (Chinese) "beautiful; swallow." Traditionally combined with another name.

Yancey: (French) "Englishman."
Also: **Yancy.**

Yarden: (Hebrew) "to flow down," as in the longest river in Israel, which flows north to south. The English name is Jordan.
Also: **Yardena, Yardenya.**

Yasmin, Yasmine: *see* Jasmine.

Yates, Yeats: (Irish) "dweller by the gate." The name honors the Irish poet William Butler Yeats.

Yedda: (Old English) "to sing."

Yelena: Russian form of Helen.

Yetta: (Teutonic) "mistress of the house."

Yin: (Chinese) "green grass; shade; musical sound." Traditionally combined with a second name.

Ying: (Chinese) "warbler; cherry; jade; welcome." Traditionally combined with a second name.

Yoki: (American Indian) "bluebird on the mesa."

Yoko: (yo-koh) (Japanese) "sun, child." Yoko Ono, musician, artist.

Yolande: (Spanish) "violet flower." Yolande Betbeze, Miss America.
Also: **Eolande, Iolanthe, Yolanda.**

Ysabel: variant of Isabel.

Yuki: (YOO-kee) (Japanese) "snow; happiness."
Also: **Yukiko.**

Yuma: an American Indian tribe name and place name.

Yuriko: (Japanese) "lily."
Also: **Yuri.**

Yvelisse: combination of Yvette and Lisa.
Also: **Ivelisse.**

Yvette: *see* Yvonne.

Yvonne: (French) "the archer."
Also: **Ivonne, Von, Vonnie, Yvette.**

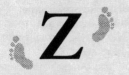

Zabrina: (Anglo-Saxon) "of the nobility."
Also: **Brina, Zabrine.**

Zada: (Arabic) "lucky one."
Also: **Zaida.**

Zahra: (Arabic/Swahili) "beautiful flower."
Also: **Zahara, Zari.**

Zakiya: (Swahili) "intelligent."

Zaltana: (American Indian) "high mountain."

Zandra: form of Alexandra. Zandra Rhodes, fashion designer.

Zara: (Hebrew) "dawn."
Also: **Zarah.**

Zarina: (Swahili) "golden."

Zea: (Latin) a kind of grain.

Zebada: (Hebrew) "gift of the Lord." Feminine of Zebadiah.
Also: **Zeba.**

Zelda: a form of Griselda. Zelda Fitzgerald, writer and wife of F. Scott Fitzgerald.

Zena: (Greek) "hospitable." (Arabic) "beautiful ornament."
Also: **Zeena, Zenia.**

Zenobia: (Greek) "having life from Jupiter."

Zephyra: (Greek) "the West Wind."
Also: **Zephra.**

Zera: (Hebrew) "seeds."

Zerlina: (Teutonic) "serene and beautiful." A principal character in Mozart's opera *Don Giovanni.*
Also: **Zerla, Zerline.**

Zeta: (Greek) the 6th letter of the Greek alphabet.

Zeva: (Greek) "sword."

Zhi: (Chinese) "iris; orchid." Traditionally combined with a second name.

Zilla: (Hebrew) "shadow."
Also: **Zillah.**

Zilpha: "distillation." Biblical: a slave who became the mother of Gad and Acher, from whom 2 of the 12 tribes of Israel descended.
Also: **Zilpah.**

Zina: (Swahili) "beauty." Zina Garrison Jackson, tennis player.

Zinah: (Hebrew) "abundance."
Also: **Zina.**

Zinaida: (Greek) "daughter of Zeus."

Zinnia: a flower name.

Zipporah: (Hebrew) "bird."
Also: **Ceporah, Tippi, Tippie, Tsiporah, Zippora.**

Zita: (Italian) "child." A 13th-century Tuscan saint. Also a diminutive of Rosita, Theresa.

Zmorah: (Zmoh-RAH) (Hebrew) "a branch or vine."

Zoe: (Greek) "life." Zoe Akins, Pulitzer prize–winning playwright.
Also: **Zoey, Zowie.**

Zoebelle: (Greek) "beautiful life."

Zofia: Polish form of Sophia.

Zola: surname of the French writer Emile Zola (1840–1902).

Zona: (Latin) "a girdle." Zona Gale, first woman to win the Pulitzer prize for drama.

Zora: (Latin) "dawn." Zora Neale Hurston, writer, anthropologist (1901–1960). Also: **Zorah, Zorana, Zorina.**

Zowie: *see* Zoe.

Zuhura: (Arabic) "brightness."

Zuleika: (Arabic) "fair."

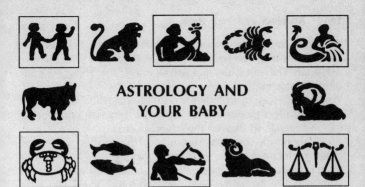

ASTROLOGY AND YOUR BABY

Although most people believe astrology is nothing more than superstition, it has nevertheless maintained a popular following. In this country an estimated $1 billion is spent annually on astrology by a diverse group, ranging from Wall Street brokers to former First Lady Nancy Reagan, who scheduled major presidential events according to astrological forecasts.

Astrological advice, or horoscopes, for the 12 birth signs continue to be a regular feature in newspapers, and new books on the subject are published and sold in big numbers every year. With the advent of computer technology, the mathematical computations for horoscopes can now be accomplished in minutes, and astrological services are readily available via the Internet.

The zodiac is an ancient star chart that was devised 2,000 years ago by astrologers who sought to track the movement of the sun. They divided the year into 12 equal parts, which correspond to 12 constellations. The concept was based on the notion that the sun passes through the 12 constellations over the course of a year. An individual's destiny was determined by the position of all the heavenly bodies at the exact time of his birth.

Modern astronomy challenges key aspects of this ancient belief system. We now know that the amount of time the sun spends in each constellation varies from a week in Scorpio to more than a month in Virgo, Taurus, and Pisces. In addition, the dates for the signs are no longer accurate, because the Earth's axis has changed, shifting the alignment with the star calendar. Therefore, declare astronomers, the zodiac is constantly changing.

Nevertheless, astrologers contend that this information does not affect their work and say that they will continue to use the zodiac in making their predictions.

Modern science notwithstanding, the zodiac will most likely maintain a place in popular culture. No matter your level of belief, or skepticism, it's just plain fun to speculate on your child's personality, behavior, and future life. That's why you'll often find an astrology section in modern baby-name books, including this one.

Children Born Under the Sign of

ARIES
March 21–April 20

Birthstone: Diamond
Flower: Sweet Pea
Color: Brilliant Red

As parents of Aries children, you may become prematurely gray worrying about what hair-raising stunt they will try next, whether their last bump will subside before they raise another, and whether any head can be injured as many times as theirs and still function properly. In Aries children, you will have a bundle of energy, enthusiasm, and dynamic power—courtesy of Mars (their ruler)—ready to explode at the slightest provocation. Their vitality is so abundant that they must remain perpetually busy, and whatever they choose to do usually involves physical activity.

They are born leaders, and it's best to let them get to the head of the class. They have the potential for recklessness, and when an idea occurs to them—and those born under the sign of Aries are constantly confronting themselves with new ones—they seldom stop to consider the consequences of their action.

Aside from the physical restraint that Aries children need, they must be taught moderation in personal conduct, in speech, and in their personal outlook upon life. Above all else, try to teach them to see each job through to completion and not to scatter their enthusiasm over a multitude of projects. Be aware, however, of your Aries' sensitive core, and never scold so harshly as to break his admirable spirit.

The bold Aries persona is tempered by demonstrative and idealistic qualities. They are generous with affection and without hesitation will come to the aid of the less fortunate or those who have suffered injustice.

If you can hang on for the ride, Aries will take you along on what will no doubt be an interesting life.

Notable people born under the sign of Aries:

Warren Beatty, actor, director—March 30
Marlon Brando, actor—April 3
Cesar Chavez, labor activist—March 31
Francis Ford Coppola, film director—April 7
Aretha Franklin, singer—March 25
Jane Goodall, ethologist—April 3
Thomas Jefferson, 3rd U.S. President—April 2
Akira Kurosawa, film director—March 23
Clare Boothe Luce, writer, U.S. ambassador—April 10
Reba McEntire, country singer—March 28
Sandra Day O'Connor, Supreme Court Justice—March 26
Stephen Sondheim, lyricist—March 22
James Watson, Nobel biochemist—April 6
Eudora Welty, author—April 13
Lanford Wilson, dramatist—April 13

Children Born Under the Sign of
TAURUS
April 21–May 21

Birthstone: Emerald
Flower: Lily-of-the-Valley
Colors: Red-Orange, Yellow

You will find that Taurus children are never carried away by wild enthusiasms, nor will they dash away to follow any leader who would be accepted by less stable and centered children. They resemble the patient bull, who must be annoyed and tormented before aroused to anger. But, as you may know, once a bull decides to fight, he makes a thorough and complete job of it. Taurus children do the same.

Taurus children will avoid conflicts; their nature is fundamentally gentle. As their parent, you may seldom see any display of anger or temper. If their temper is aroused, however, you will never forget it, for under these conditions, they are not only furious and headstrong, but stubborn in yielding to the opinion or authority of others. Still, on the whole they will give you far less worry than most other children. Your little bull loves affection, and will seize every opportunity to cuddle in your lap. Use the same loving manner when giving parental guidance, for harsh discipline will only get his or her back up. In school and other endeavors Taurus will succeed at a quiet, steady pace, learning in his or her methodical way. Like Ferdinand the Bull, from the children's story, Taurus will have a unique appreciation of the beauty of nature, music, and art. Give him opportunities to explore these areas, which may lead him to a lifelong avocation.

Notable people born under the sign of Taurus:
John James Audubon, painter, naturalist—April 26
Willem de Kooning, artist—April 24
Ariel Durant, historian, author—May 10
Elizabeth II, queen of England—April 21
Nora Ephron, film director, writer—May 19
Ella Fitzgerald, singer—April 25
Pancho Gonzales, tennis player—May 9
Martha Graham, dancer, choreographer—May 11
Isabella I, queen of Castile—April 22
Zubin Mehta, conductor—April 29
Golda Meir, prime minister of Israel—May 3
Jack Nicholson, actor—April 28
I. M. Pei, architect—April 26
Eva Perón, Argentine political figure—May 7
Jacob Riis, social reformer—May 3
Barbra Streisand, entertainer—April 24

Children Born Under the Sign of

GEMINI

May 22–June 21

Birthstone: Pearl
Flower: Rose
Color: Violet

Only the parents of twins can appreciate the challenge that falls to the parents of Gemini children. For Gemini is the sign of the twins, and Gemini children may seem at times to be two people in one. A Gemini baby is "all over the place"—both physically and mentally, they seem to be going in all directions at once.

They are bright and alert, and extremely inquisitive. They will keep you hopping through the early years, and you will be tempted to stifle that high energy, if only to give everyone a rest. But you may end up frustrating yourselves and the little Gemini, who cannot completely defy her inherent high-strung nature.

Since Mercury governs the vocal chords, Gemini will impress you with her facility for language. Before she has words she will communicate from her crib, and in an astonishing range of volume. In school, she will excel in reading and composition. Her active curiosity will have her doing well in other subjects, but at the same time allow her to be easily distracted in the classroom.

Part of the constant questioning of these children is due to an actual desire for information, for they are always very bright, but their curiosity is rather superficial. They want to know something about everything that happens to cross their path, but they may not persist in one line of thought for very long. The most valuable lesson parents can teach their busy

Gemini is to stick to one thing at a time. Make sure to give them a physical outlet for their nervous energy; this will help their concentration skills and ensure their good health.

Notable people born under the sign of Gemini:

Margaret Bourke-White, photographer—June 14
Rachel Carson, writer—May 27
Jacques Cousteau—marine biologist, June 11
Bob Dylan, singer—May 24
Clint Eastwood, actor, director—May 31
Allen Ginsberg, poet—June 3
Steffi Graf, tennis player—June 14
Katharine Graham, owner, *Washington Post*—June 16
John F. Kennedy, 35th U.S. President—May 29
Henry Kissinger, U.S. secretary of state—May 27
Ludwig Mies van der Rohe, architect—May 27
Norman Vincent Peale, clergyman—May 31
Sally Ride, astronaut—May 26
Harriet Beecher Stowe, author, social reformer—June 14
Walt Whitman, poet—May 31
Frank Lloyd Wright, architect—June 8

Children Born Under the Sign of

CANCER

June 22–July 23

Birthstone: Ruby
Flower: Lily
Colors: Delicate Greens

These children have an extremely sensitive nature. From their infancy, they are highly aware of their environment and are greatly affected by it. Their emotional profile is equally sensitive, and you may see a wide range of moods over the course of a day.

Needless to say, early childhood can be a critical period for such tender souls. Care should be taken to cultivate feelings of acceptance and security, which are necessary to the Cancer child's well-being. Later on, try to avoid Spartan methods of discipline, for Cancer children are better ruled by love and encouragement, and will not do their best in an atmosphere of disapproval.

Their mild-mannered nature will make them well-received by others. And being so sensitive, they are highly astute, which also makes them good with people. Their unselfish nature, however, may cause others to frequently impose upon them. While they are not inclined toward aggressiveness, they will express the crab's tenacity and determination when they have been aroused to defend their rights. Cancer children have a true spirit of patriotism and pride in their country and their home. You will hear them telling their playmates that their family is the best, for that's the way they feel about their loved ones. They will appreciate their home and spend more time in it than most other children. Their strong attachment to mother and home usually continues throughout life.

World events make a profound impression on these children, who generally are very much in tune with what's going on. They will have a strong appreciation of history, and will excel in the subject in school. Not surprisingly, they will have a natural inclination to travel. Such experiences will only serve to enhance their academic education.

Notable people born under the sign of Cancer:
Arthur Ashe, tennis player—July 10
Mary McLeod Bethune, educator—July 10
Van Cliburn, pianist—July 12
Mary Baker Eddy, religious leader—July 16
Harrison Ford, actor—July 13
John Glenn, astronaut, politician—July 18
Ernest Hemingway, author—July 21
Frida Kahlo, artist—July 6
Helen Keller, writer, advocate for the physically challenged—June 27
Carl Lewis, track star—July 1
Pablo Neruda, poet—July 12
Ellison Onizuka, astronaut—June 24
Joseph Papp, theatre director/producer—June 22
Isaac Stern, violinist—July 21
Meryl Streep, actress—June 22
Billy Wilder, film director—June 22

Children Born Under the Sign of
LEO
July 24–August 23

Birthstone: Peridot
Flower: Gladiolus
Color: Orange

These children want to be the center of attention—favorable attention, of course. They thrive on adulation; they demand praise for all that they do, and they will do a surprising amount with the stimulus of "That's fine. You are wonderful." They are more responsive to love and tenderness than to punishment, and care should be taken not to rein them in too harshly.

One of the greatest attributes of a Leo is his natural facility for leadership. This will be evident from a very early age and may frustrate parents, who cannot cope with what may appear to be simple tyranny. Hard as it may seem, do not crush this hallmark of the Leo personality, which will serve him so well later in life.

While they tend to take charge, they are basically big-hearted people who are more strongly motivated by love than selfishness. When put to the test, no sacrifice is too great for them to make on behalf of a loved one. Their magnanimous nature also makes them quick to forgive. They seldom have enemies, for their hearts have no room for hate.

The school-age Leo will naturally assert himself in the classroom, which may ensure success or put him at odds with the teacher. He is intelligent and can be highly creative, but he will continue to require praise and encouragement in order for him to fulfill his potential.

Notable people born under the sign of Leo:
Bella Abzug, congresswoman—July 24
Neil Armstrong, astronaut—August 5
Julia Child, author, television personality—August 15
Robert De Niro, actor—August 17
Thomas Eakins, painter—July 25
Amelia Earhart, aviatrix—July 24
Milton Friedman, economist—July 31
Dustin Hoffman, actor—August 8
Whitney Houston, singer—August 9
Carl Jung, psychologist—July 26
Louis Leakey, archaeologist, anthropologist—August 7
Henry Moore, sculptor—July 30
Jacqueline Bouvier Kennedy Onassis, First Lady of the U.S.—July 28
Robert Redford, actor, director—August 18
Pat Schroeder, congresswoman—July 30

Children Born Under the Sign of

VIRGO
August 24–September 23

Birthstone: Sapphire
Flower: Aster
Color: Dark Violet

Virgo children, above all others, should be given every opportunity for a thorough and complete education. They have an inherent thirst for knowledge, which is complemented by a methodical and practical disposition.

These children may take interest in a variety of subjects and will study for the sheer pleasure of learning. They make high grades in school, and their cooperative natures make them favorites with their teachers. At home parents will find Virgos just as cooperative. Order and routine are natural and pleasing to them, and you will seldom complain that they don't pick up their clothes or keep their rooms in order. On the other hand, don't be surprised if they hold everyone else to the same standard of neatness.

While they are good students, they are less interested in becoming class president, and will not assert themselves socially. Teach them not to be too critical of others, and they will come to understand the value of friendships. They should also learn not to be too hard on themselves, for they have a tendency for perfectionism.

While they may appear almost self-sufficient, make sure to attend to your Virgo's emotional needs, offering plenty of physical affection. Actively encourage fantasy and make-believe play with your little realist to give her some balance.

Notable people born under the sign of Virgo:
Jane Addams, social reformer—September 6
Ingrid Bergman, actress—August 29
Leonard Bernstein, conductor, composer—August 25
Joyce Brothers, psychologist—September 20
Ray Charles, singer—September 23
Agatha Christie, writer—September 15
Jimmy Connors, tennis player—September 9
Stephen Jay Gould, paleontologist—September 10
Daniel K. Inouye, Senator—September 7
Jeremy Irons, actor—September 19
Maria Montessori, educator—August 31
Jessye Norman, opera singer—September 15
Charlie Parker, jazz musician—August 29
Bruce Springsteen, singer—September 23
Mother Teresa, humanitarian—August 27

Children Born Under the Sign of
LIBRA
September 24–October 23

Birthstone: Opal
Flowers: Calendula, Cosmos
Color: Yellow

These children show artistic tendencies at an early age. They are graceful and attractive when compared with children of other signs. They are the ones who are called upon by a fond teacher to sing a solo in recital or draw the cover of the school magazine. There is a reason for this popularity beyond their considerable artistic abilities. They are extremely easy to get along with; and in association with children of stronger will, count on them to let others have their way in order to keep the peace.

Their easygoing nature, however, could hamper future development, for above everything else, they need to develop willpower—the will to stick to whatever they start until they have made a success of it. Early in life, show them that success in any field is one-third talent and two-thirds perseverance. In other words, don't let them be dilettantes who fritter away their latent abilities.

Librans are lovable and will give parents little trouble. However, parent and child may at times become frustrated with Libra's difficulty in making decisions. This is part of her nature; after all, she lives by the sign of the scales and is constantly trying to achieve balance. Be patient and don't rush her; instead, teach her decision-making skills, and she'll soon learn to get on with it.

In important matters, Libra generally makes the right choice, for she is very concerned with fairness. Her sense of balance allows young Libra the perspective to consider both sides of an issue. Like the scales, Libra can swing to extremes in terms of mood and activity. Those around her will just have to accommodate these changes until Libra attains the peaceful, harmonious balance that she seeks.

Notable people born under the sign of Libra:
Bruce Catton, historian, author—October 8
Robert Coles, child psychiatrist—October 12
Michael Crichton, author—October 23
Jim Henson, "Muppets" creator—September 24
John Lennon, singer, songwriter—October 9
Doris Lessing, author—October 22
Maya Lin, architect—October 5
Martina Navratilova, tennis player—October 10
Eleanor Roosevelt, U.N. ambassador—October 11
Susan Sarandon, actress—October 4
Margaret Thatcher, British prime minister—October 13
Gore Vidal, author—October 3
Grete Waitz, champion long-distance runner—October 1
Barbara Walters, broadcaster—September 25
Wendy Wasserstein, dramatist—October 18

Children Born Under the Sign of
SCORPIO
October 24–November 22

Birthstone: Topaz
Flower: Chrysanthemum
Color: Deep Red

There should be no doubt about it—parents will find a challenging job ahead of them if their child is born under the sign of the Scorpion. From infancy, Scorpio children will demonstrate their dynamic personalities, which on occasion may erupt explosively. These are powerful people, gifted with intelligence and strong wills.

Moderation is practically unknown to these children; and half measures, to them, are worse than none. They are either all for something or someone or so bitterly opposed that no force or argument can sway them. They are unafraid of confrontation and will take on any challenge. They are intensely loyal to friends and family, and will take up their cause in addition to their own. They can be blunt in speech and display a quick temper, so it is essential in early life to take them in hand and teach them self-control and respect for others. This will not be an easy task, for they have an unusual amount of determination and do not obey without knowing the reason for doing so. Reason with them and avoid a condescending manner, and you will find them responsive and loyal. The more straightforward you are in your relations with them, the more they will respect and learn from you.

Scorpios have physical energy in proportion to their strong personalities. These robust children are constantly on the move, and they possess great recuperative powers, recovering quickly from illness.

With gentle guidance, Scorpio will be successful in life, and parents will be rewarded to see his abundant energy and passion help him achieve his goals.

Notable people born under the sign of Scorpio:
Abigail Adams, wife and mother of two U.S. Presidents—November 11
Jane Alexander, actress, chair, National Endowment for the Arts—October 28
Marie Curie, scientist—November 7
Jodie Foster, actress, director—November 19
Indira Gandhi, prime minister of India—November 19
Bill Gates, chairman, Microsoft—October 28
Katharine Hepburn, actress—November 8
C. S. Lewis, author—November 29
Mike Nichols, film director—November 6
Isamu Noguchi, sculptor—November 17
Georgia O'Keeffe, artist—November 15
Theodore Roosevelt, 26th U.S. President—November 27
Carl Sagan, scientist—November 9
Martin Scorsese, film director—November 17
Ted Turner, businessman—November 19
Kurt Vonnegut, author—November 11

Children Born Under the Sign of
SAGITTARIUS
November 23–December 21

Birthstone: Turquoise
Flower: Narcissus
Colors: Deep Blue, Purple

These children are not only hopeful and trusting, but gay and light of heart. Truthfulness and a natural lack of selfishness are other fine qualities that may be expected of them. They are idealistic and strong of faith, and often form strong spiritual inclinations. You might be wise to teach them, before they learn from painful experience, that they are not to believe all that they hear, as their own truthful nature makes them believe that everyone they encounter will be just as honest.

They judge others by their own high standards, and they lack suspiciousness because they have none of the qualities which arouse it in themselves. In your own relations with them, show appreciation of their trustworthiness by giving them all possible freedom. They will have more than the usual amount of childish curiosity, and they will not only ask many questions but may be very analytical and critical of those around them. As parent, your directives will constantly be subject to their scrutiny, and their questioning will become increasingly sophisticated as they mature. Whatever you do, don't lie, as their honest natures deserve to be rewarded in kind.

Sagittarus children love the outdoors and active sports. Try to see to it that they are never without pets of some kind, for they are born animal-lovers and will learn much from taking care of them. In the matter of education, let them follow their own inclinations, for their ambitions may range from the ministry to law. Again, trust the aim of your little archer, and she will happily find her mark in life.

Notable people born under the sign of Sagittarius:

Dave Brubeck, jazz musician—December 6
Lane Bryant, businesswoman—December 1
Maria Callas, opera singer—December 4
Shirley Chisholm, congresswoman—November 30
Sir Winston Churchill, British prime minister—November 30
Walt Disney, entertainment pioneer—December 5
Chris Evert, tennis player—December 21
Joe DiMaggio, baseball player—November 25
John Malkovich, actor—December 19
David Mamet, dramatist—November 30
Mary, Queen of Scots—December 8
Margaret Mead, anthropologist—December 16
Charles Schulz, cartoonist—November 26
Steven Spielberg, film director—December 18
Mark Twain, writer—November 30

Children Born Under the Sign of

CAPRICORN
December 22–January 20

Birthstone: Garnet
Flower: Carnation
Color: Deep Blue

At first glance, a Capricorn will strike you as less flashy than those born under other signs; quiet and unobtrusive, he appears to trod a straight-and-narrow path. He respects authority and obeys social conventions, and will acquiesce to the wishes of more assertive people. But, of course, there's more to him than meets the eye. Behind the quiet demeanor is an active, ambitious mind, backed by a remarkably strong will.

From infancy Capricorns seem mature beyond their years, and their agreeable natures make for relatively easy parenting. However, they have definite likes and dislikes, which they will make known to you. You need not worry about how your Capricorn will handle schoolwork, for they are inclined to study hard and put into practical use the knowledge that they gain. Not infrequently, you will find them interested in some line of study leading to a trade or a profession. They will attain positions of leadership as others recognize and reward their responsible nature. Don't, however, expect them to be hail-fellows-well-met. They will never aspire to be cheerleaders. If they have anything to do with the team, it will probably be as business managers, not star players.

Don't try to defy their nature and "draw them out of their shell," or they may become self-conscious and more solitary. They have mental resources within themselves and often prefer their own company to that of other children.

Saturn's influence as ruler of Capricorn bestows the valuable qualities of efficiency, levelheadedness, and conscientiousness to these children, which will serve them well as they make their own, unique way in the world.

Notable people born under the sign of Capricorn:
Alvin Ailey, dancer, choreographer—January 5
Muhammad Ali, boxer—January 18
Elizabeth Arden, businesswoman—December 31
Kevin Costner, actor, director—January 18
E. L. Doctorow, author—January 6
Benjamin Franklin, statesman—December 25
Marilyn Horne, opera singer—January 16
Zora Neale Hurston, writer—January 7
Diane Keaton, actress—January 5
Martin Luther King, civil rights leader—January 15
Nancy Lopez, golfer—January 6
Sir Isaac Newton, scientist—December 27
Elvis Presley, singer—January 8
Anwar Sadat, Egyptian president—December 25
J. D. Salinger, author—January 1
Albert Schweitzer, philosopher, medical missionary—January 14

Children Born Under the Sign of

AQUARIUS
January 21–February 19

Birthstone: Amethyst
Flower: Violet
Color: Light Blue

These children are social creatures. Companionships are important to all Aquarians, and throughout their lives they will be blessed with multitudes of friends. As parent, you will be wise to make companions of them rather than assume the role of stern master, for these children do not need strict discipline and are generally more obedient to your wishes than children of most other signs. In their search for companionship, they will seek out those who are older than they are. They possess above-average intelligence for their age, and since they are agreeable companions, they risk being spoiled with too much attention and allowed too many privileges for their years.

Their many friendships tend to be lasting ones, due to Aquarian's constant nature. This fixed point of view may result in a certain degree of stubbornness, which is most effectively handled with affection and reason.

Parents should actively encourage physical, outdoor activity, since Aquarians have a tendency to prefer the indoors and more intellectual pursuits. They will be eager and competent students; philosophy, science, and literature will be particular areas of interest. There is frequently inventive ability along scientific lines, and they will also find great interest in humanitarian work. These children rarely lead dull lives.

Notable people born under the sign of Aquarius:
Susan B. Anthony, women's suffragist—February 15
Corazon Aquino, president of the Philippines—January 25
Placido Domingo, opera singer—January 21
Thomas Edison, inventor—February 11
Betty Friedan, writer, feminist—February 4
Michael Jordan, basketball player—February 17
Abraham Lincoln, 16th U.S. President—February 12
Charles Lindbergh, aviator—February 2
Toni Morrison, author—February 18
Paul Newman, actor—January 26
Jackson Pollock, artist—January 28
Amy Tan, author—February 19
Barbara Tuchman, historian—January 30
Alice Walker, author—February 9
Simone Weil, philosopher—February 3
Oprah Winfrey, television personality—January 29

Children Born Under the Sign of
PISCES
February 20–March 20

Birthstone: Aquamarine
Flower: Jonquil
Color: Dark Purple

Those born under the watery sign of the fish do seem otherworldly at times, for these are the dreamers of the zodiac. They possess incredible imaginative powers and, if given the structure and guidance they need, will find great success in the arts, particularly acting.

Pisces is a negative sign, which makes these children extremely sensitive to outside influences, so parents should take care to avoid unfavorable ones until they are old enough to judge right from wrong. Overall, Pisceans require a restraining influence to balance their freewheeling, dreamy-eyed tendencies. This is especially important in early childhood.

They are capable of acquiring a good education, though they may not always fit in with standard educational methods. But teachers will always find them agreeable and pliant components in the classroom. At home impose some focus and structure in their lives, which will help balance their daydreaming ways. Tasks or chores will also help ground them with a sense of responsibility.

Take care not to go too far in correcting these free, artistic spirits. As parent you may need to protect the Piscean's dreams from the cold practicality of society-at-large, until he can fulfill them.

Notable people born under the sign of Pisces:
Ansel Adams, photographer—February 20
Mario Andretti, race car driver—February 28
Alexander Graham Bell, inventor—March 3
Glenn Close, actress—March 19
Albert Einstein, scientist—March 14
Ralph Ellison, author—March 1
Ruth Bader Ginsburg, Supreme Court justice—March 15
John Irving, author—March 2
Quincy Jones, musician, producer—March 14
Spike Lee, film director—March 20
Mary Ellen Mark, photojournalist—March 20
Linus Pauling, chemist—February 28
Elizabeth Taylor, actress—February 27
Valentina Tereshkova, first woman to travel in space—March 6
John Updike, author—March 18
George Washington, 1st U.S. President—February 22

SUGGESTIONS FOR FURTHER READING

Carpenter, Humphrey and Mari Prichard. *The Oxford Companion to Children's Literature.* New York: Oxford University Press, 1984.

Carr, Ian. *Jazz: The Essential Companion.* New York: Prentice Hall Press, 1987.

Coggins, Richard. *Who's Who in the Bible.* Totowa, N.J.: Barnes & Noble Books, 1981.

Cresswell, Julia. *Tuttle Dictionary of First Names.* Boston: Charles E. Tuttle Company, 1990.

Dunkling, Leslie and William Gosling. *The New American Dictionary of Baby Names.* New York: Penguin Books, 1985.

Ellefson, Connie Lockhart. *The Melting Pot Book of Baby Names.* White Hall, Va.: Betterway Publications, Inc., 1987.

von Engelin, O. D. *The Story Key to Geographic Names.* New York: D. Appleton and Company, 1924.

Ewen, David. *American Songwriters.* New York: H. W. Wilson Co., 1987.

Grzebieniowski, Tadeuz. *Langenscheidt's Pocket Polish Dictionary.* 1985.

Kolatch, Alfred J. *Dictionary of First Names.* Middle Village, N.Y.: Jonathan David Publishers, 1980.

Laing, Hardy and Dave. *Encyclopedia of Rock.* New York: Schirmer Books, 1988.

Loughead, Flora Haines. *Dictionary of Given Names.* Glendale, Ca.: Arthur H. Clark Company, 1974.

MacLysaght, Edward. *The Surnames of Ireland.* Shannon, Ireland: Irish University Press, 1969.

Martin, Mick and Marsha Porter. *Video Movie Guide 1996.* New York: Ballantine Books, 1995.

Pringle, David. *Imaginary People: A Who's Who of Modern Fictional Characters.* New York: Pharos Books, 1987.

Pukui, Mary Kawena and Samuel H. Elbert. *Hawaiian-English Dictionary.* Honolulu: University of Hawaii Press, 1957.

Sanchez, Nellie Van de Grift. *Spanish and Indian Place Names of California: Their Meaning and Their Romance.* San Francisco: A. M. Robertson, 1930.

Shan, Lin. *Name Your Baby in Chinese.* Union City, Ca.: Heian International, Inc., 1988.

Sleigh, Linwood and Charles Johnson. *The Book of Boys' Names.* New York: Thomas Y. Crowell, 1962.

Smith, Elsdon C. *Dictionary of American Family Names.* New York: Harper & Row Publishers, 1956.

Stewart, George R. *American Given Names.* New York: Oxford University Press, 1979.

Stewart, Julia. *African Names.* New York: Carol Publishing Group, 1993.

Telgen, Diane and Jim Kamp, Editors. *Notable Hispanic American Women.* Detroit: Gale Research, Inc., 1993.

Thomas, Nicholas, Editor. *International Dictionary of Films and Filmmakers: Directors 2nd Edition.* Chicago: St. James Press, 1991.

Uwate, Aiko Nishi. *Japanese Names for Babies.* Los Angeles: 1982.

York, William. *Who's Who in Rock Music.* New York: Charles Scribner's Sons, 1982.

KATHY ISHIZUKA
is a freelance writer. She lives in
New York City with her family.